Progress in Public Health

Edited by

Gabriel Scally
Regional Director of Public Health, S & W Regional Office, NHS Executive, Bristol

With Foreword by
Sir Kenneth Calman
Chief Medical Officer, England

FINANCIAL TIMES
Healthcare

FT HEALTHCARE
a Division of Pearson Professional Ltd
Maple House, 149 Tottenham Court Road,
London W1P 9LL, UK
Telephone: +44 (0)171 896 2424
Fax: +44 (0)171 896 2449
http://www.fthealthcare.com

First published 1997

A catalogue record for this book is available from
the British Library

ISBN 0-443-05938-1

Publisher: Mark Lane
Project Manager: Kate Lodge, Hertford

Typeset by Saxon Graphics Ltd., Derby

Printed and bound in Great Britain by
Antony Rowe Ltd, Chippenham, Wiltshire

Contents

List of Figures

Contributors

John Ashton
Regional Director of Public Health, N & W Regional Office, NHS Executive, Warrington

Kay Beaumont
Team Manager, Southwark Social Services, Maudsley Hospital, London

Yaov Ben-Shlomo
Department of Social Medicine, University of Bristol

David Benton
Regional Director of Nursing, Northern and Yorkshire Region and Professor of Nursing, University of Northumbria at Newcastle

Neil Boot
Health Promotion Advisor, Plymouth

David Briggs
Director of the Nene Centre for Research, Nene College, Boughton, Northampton

George Davey Smith
Department of Social Medicine, University of Bristol

Liam Donaldson
Regional Director/Regional Director of Public Health. Northern & Yorkshire Regional Office, Durham, and Professor of Applied Epidemiology, University of Newcastle upon Tyne

Robin Downie
Department of Philosophy, The University of Glasgow

Paul Elliott
Head of Department, Department of Epidemiology and Public Health Medicine, School of Medicine at St Mary's, London

John Fox
Chief Medical Statistician, National Office of Statistics

Hilary Guite
Consultant Public Health Medicine, Bromley Health, Hayes, Kent and Research Fellow, Community Division, Kings School of Medicine and Dentistry, London

David J Hunter
Professor of Health Policy and Management, and Director of the Nuffield Institute for Health, University of Leeds

Ian Jones
Medical Director, Centre for Health and Social Research, Glenrothes, Fife

Debra Lapthorne
Team Leader, Plymouth

Martin McKee
Professor of European Public Health, London School of Hygiene and Tropical Medicine

Jane Macnaughton
Department of General Practice, University of Glasgow

Moira Maconachie
Senior Research Fellow, Department of Sociology, University of Plymouth/Public Health Team

Klim McPherson
Health Promotion Sciences Unit, Department of Public Health & Policy, London School of Hygiene and Tropical Medicine

Ruairidh Milne
Senior Lecturer in Public Health Medicine, Wessex Institute for Health Services Research and Development, Southampton University

Elias Mossialos
Senior Research Fellow, London School of Economics and Political Science

J. A. Muir Gray
Director of R&D, Anglia and Oxford Region, Oxford

Georgina Radford
Director of Public Health, S & W Devon HA, Dartington, Devon

Gabriel Scally
Regional Director of Public Health, S & W Regional Office, NHS Executive, Bristol

Rosalind Stanwell Smith
Consultant Epidemiologist, Communicable Disease Surveillance Centre, London

Andrew Stevens
The Medical School, University of Birmingham

Graham Thornicroft
Professor of Community Psychiatry, Institute of Psychiatry and Director of PRiSM

Drew Walker
Director of Public Health, Ayshire and Arran Health Board

Patrick Wall
Consultant, Communicable Disease Surveillance Centre, London

Foreword

In writing a foreword the author needs to capture the spirit of the book in question and set both the scene and the tone. A key word is usually necessary, and this is generally dictated by the title. In this case the choice was relatively easy, and the important word is 'progress'. In definitional terms this concerns forward movement and advance. It indicates that something has changed and that this is for the better. This book therefore sets out to look at progress in public health.

It is convenient, in this case, to use a very broad definition of public health and what is striking is just how much progress has been made. It has not generated the same excitement as gene therapy or cardiac transplantation, yet the progress is there and it affects us all. Changing the health of a population takes time and sustained effort. Progress must occur at all levels, in government, at community level and with individuals. In making progress, in effecting change, a wide range of people need to be involved. In addition to the professional staff, doctors, nurses, economists, epidemiologists, environmental scientists, behavioural psychologists, educationalists and many others, there is a need to involve politicians, specialist groups, voluntary organisations, trade unions and managers in the process. Progress can only be made if they all work together to a common goal, improving the health of the public.

The book discusses areas where progress has occurred and where progress needs to occur. Inequalities, deprivation and community development are all topics of the highest importance. Managing public health better will also lead to a greater progress based on a clear vision for the new millennium. More detailed topics, such as small area statistics, screening and communicable disease control show just what has changed over the years. Central to this has been greater involvement of the public in making choices and setting goals. The issues are difficult, which makes it even more important that the public are seen to be part of the process and are linked with any progress made.

At the heart of making progress is the value system which is espoused by those who make decisions or who implement programmes to improve the public health. These values set the agenda and are closely linked to the ethical dimensions and problems discussed in the book. The overall objective is to improve the common weal. Progress has been made but must continue to be made. This book takes us a step in that direction.

KENNETH C CALMAN
June 1997

List of Abbreviations

ACP	American College of Physicians
AEA	Atomic Energy Authority
AIDS	Acquired Immuno Deficiency Syndrome
AMA	Association of Metropolitan Authorities
ASW	Approved Social Worker
APHA	American Public Health Association
ARIF	Aggressive Research Intelligence Facility
BMA	British Medical Association
BMJ	British Medical Journal
BOD	Biological Oxygen Demand
BSE	Bovine Spongiform Encephalopathy
CASP	Critical Appraisal Skills Programme
CESDI	Confidential Enquiry into Stillbirths and Deaths in Infancy
CHD	Coronary Heart Disease
CJD	Creutzfeldt–Jacob Disease
CMHT	Community Mental Health Team
CMO	Chief Medical Officer
CPA	Care Programme Approach
CPN	Care Programme Nurse
CRD	Centre for Reviews and Dissemination
CSAG	Clinical Standard Advisory Group
CT	Computerised Tomography
DALY	Disability Adjusted Life Years
DARE	Database of Abstracts of Reviews and Effectiveness
DEC	Development and Evaluation Centre
DGM	District General Manager
DHA	District Health Authority

DPH	Director of Public Health
DSS	Department of Social Security
DoH	Department of Health
EBM	Evidence-Based Medicine
EC	Economic Community
ECG	Electrocardiogram
E.coli	*Escherichia coli*
EEG	Electroencephalogram
EHE	Enterohaemorrhagic E.coli
EU	European Union
EUN	Enhanced Urban Network
EUPHA	European Public Health Association
E&W	England and Wales
FPHM	Faculty of Public Health Medicine
GEARS	Getting Easier Access to Reviews
GIS	Geographical Information System
GRiPP	Getting Research into Practice and Purchasing
GRO(S)	General Register Office (Scotland)
GUM	GenitoUrinary Medicine
HEDIS	Health Plan Employer Data and Information Set
HFA 2000	Health for All by the year 2000
HIV	Human Immunodeficiency Virus
HMSO	Her Majesty's Stationery Office
HoNOS	Health of the Nation Outcome Scale
HSI	Health Service Indicator
HTA	Health Technology Assessment
IDU	Intravenous Drug User
ISD	Information and Statistics Division
JAMA	Journal of the American Medical Association
JCAHO	Joint Commission on Accreditation of Health Care Organisations
LSL	Lambeth, Southwark and Lewisham
MDPHF	Mulit-Disciplinary Public Health Forum

MHA	Mental Health Act
MHR	Medical and Health Research
MINI	Mental Illness Needs Index
MRI	Magnetic Resonance Imaging
NAHAT	National Association of Health Authorities and Trusts
NHS	National Health Service
NMET	Non-Medical Education and Training
NNT	Number Needed to Treat
NRR	National Research Register
ONS	Office for National Statistics
PACE	Promoting Action on Clinical Effectiveness
PCV	Prescribed Concentration Value
PHM	Public Health Medicine
PET	Positron Emission Tomography
PrP	Prion gene
QALY	Quality Adjusted Life Year
RCGP	Royal College of General Practitioners
RCT	Randomised Controlled Trial
R&D	Research and Development
REITOX	réseau eurpéan d'information sur la toxicomanie
RHA	Regional Health Authority
SBO	Specified Bovine Offal
SBU	Swedish Council on Technology Assessment in Health Care
SEAC	Spongiform Encephalopathy Advisory Committee
SHEP	Systolic Hypertension in the Elderly Programme
SMR	Standardised Mortality Rate
SSM	Society for Social Medicine
SSPE	Subacute Sclerosing Panencephalitis
SSRI	Specific Serotinin Reuptake Inhibitor
STD	Sexually Transmitted Disease
TAPS	Team for the Assessment of Psychiatric Services
UK	United Kingdom

UNICEF	United Nations International Children's Emergency Fund
USA	United States of America
USSR	Union of Soviet Socialist Republics
VOD	Volatile Organic Compound
WHO	World Health Organisation

1. Introduction

Gabriel Scally

The desire of human communities to improve the health status of their citizens has been one of the fundamental goals of civilisation for thousands of years. Threats to health faced by early communities, particularly from epidemic diseases, led to the creation of complex systems of public health protection even in the absence of well developed theories of disease causation. Although their role and function has changed radically down the centuries the current generation of public health professionals can be justifiably proud of a lineage that can be traced back at least as far as the city physicians of ancient Greece (Rosen 1993). In 1997 the public health community in Britain celebrated the 150th anniversary of one of the important events in the history of public health, the appointment of the first Medical Officers of Health. It is likely that in due course 1997 will be remembered in its own right for the landmark creation within government of the post of Minister for Public Health.

The visionary approach taken by the World Health Organisation (WHO) in adopting the programme 'Health For All by the year 2000' (HFA 2000) inspired many of those with an interest in the public health to question contemporary practice and develop a wider and societal based approach. In his chapter John Ashton reflects on this important initiative and how it might continue to inspire and encourage beyond the year 2000. The preamble to the constitution of WHO defines health as a state of complete physical, social and mental well-being and it is this broadly based definition that lies behind HFA 2000. Although the physical and social aspects of health are home territories for public health professionals, mental health has to some extent been neglected as pointed out by Hilary Guite and her colleagues in their contribution to this book.

The challenge to public health professionals as we approach a new millennium comes from a world that is in rapid transition. The advent of mass air travel and enormously increased international trade has produced a dramatic increase in the mobility of people, products and disease. At one stage public health practitioners might have thought that, at least in the developed world, communicable disease was not only under control but also in decline. The emergence of new diseases, and new strains of old ones, has changed that view and in their chapter Pat Wall and Ros Stanwell Smith note the many challenges in communicable disease that face us now and in the future.

The same development of civilisation that has created these opportunities for travel and trade, with their attendant risks, has also placed an increasing strain on the global environment. Global warming, the destruction of forests and hedgerows, and the over-fishing of our oceans are all likely, if not checked, to have serious consequences for the health of human populations. The concern about environmental factors that was displayed in the Hippocratic treatise 'On airs, waters and places' has however not been prominent among public health professionals in recent times. The growth in public concern about local environmental hazards such as radiation and toxic chemicals has lead the development of an important strand of public health science as outlined by Paul Elliott and David Briggs in their chapter.

The rapid transition that has taken place in the world at large has been mirrored in the area of health service organisation and provision both in Britain and in Europe. The growing role of the European Union (EU) in the public health field can sometimes be overlooked. As Britain's previously insular approach to the EU gives way to a policy of active engagement, Martin McKee and Elias Mossialos in their chapter remind us of its importance to public health. The introduction of a purchaser–provider split in health services has become an accepted part of the orthodoxy of health service organisation and has in theory liberated public health professionals from direct responsibility for the management of clinical services. This is, supposedly, to their advantage as they can then concentrate on improving the health of populations for which they are responsible. The contribution that can be made to the improvement of clinical services can however potentially distract attention from the task of addressing the wider environmental and social causes of ill health such as poor housing, poverty and unemployment. The evidence of persisting, and in some case widening, inequalities in health experience amongst the population of the UK is compelling and is clearly stated in the contribution by George Davey Smith and Yoav Ben-Shlomo. The chapter by Gina Radford and her colleagues reminds us that the ability to engage effectively with deprived local communities in the struggle to improve health is key to the future of public health practice.

There can be little doubt that a re-engagement of public health practitioners with the social and environmental determinants of health is long overdue. The necessary correction in the balance of effort should not however lead to the neglect of the important contribution that can be made to health services issues. Central to public health concerns is the question of the quality of health care provided to a population. In their chapter Liam Donaldson and David Benton argue that public health skills have much to contribute to the creation of integrated strategies for improving quality. Closely related to the broad issue of quality, the topic of clinical effectiveness is one of the dominant themes of the late 1990s. As Andrew Stevens and Ruairidh Milne argue in their contribution, the clinical effectiveness agenda contains key messages for public health professionals. In particular the question of the effectiveness of screening is more than worthy of the chapter devoted to it by Muir Gray. Screening poses many challenges in the field of ethics and Robin Downie and Jane Macnaughton address this amongst other important ethical issues in their chapter.

The creation of a well-developed public health function that is capable of carrying out the wide range of tasks necessary has been one of the greatest challenges to public health professionals in the past decade. All too often the goals of 'management' are seen as divorced from public health concerns. In his chapter David Hunter develops the concept of 'public health management' as a means of avoiding the marginalisation that often befalls public health practitioners. The passion to improve the health of the people that must exist in any true public health practitioner is not, and never has been, the preserve of the medically qualified. One of the greatest tasks that faces those engaged in the public health function is to ensure that all those, from whatever professional background, who have the training and expertise to contribute to our collective efforts have the opportunity to do so. Klim McPherson and his colleagues in their chapter argue that the range of tasks requiring public health input leaves ample scope for a wide spectrum of professional groups to make their contribution, but that it is necessary to achieve parity of esteem before this united effort can be fully effective.

Although this book attempts to cover some of the areas that are important to those with an interest in the public health, any one book can never be comprehensive. It is the nature of a speciality that can potentially be concerned with every aspect of human existence that there will always be influences on health that are not dealt with adequately. The issues of gender and ethnicity are for example not considered in any substantial way amongst the chapters in this book but are of course powerful influences on health experience. What is of crucial importance is that we have an understanding of the theories that guide our approach to such important issues. This case is put firmly by Ian Jones and Drew Walker in their chapter that revisits some earlier work on the theories that underlie public health practice. Irrespective of our individual theoretical base it is however vitally important for public health professionals to identify in some collective fashion, the priorities to which we should be devoting our energy and the all too small resource at our disposal. The call for a collective approach should not mean some stifling central control but rather the creation of opportunities to inspire and support those engaged in the task of producing change. Hopefully public health practitioners will always question the accepted orthodoxy and display what George Bernard Shaw termed 'divine discontent'.

REFERENCES

Rosen G 1993 A History of Public Health. Baltimore: The John Hopkins University Press

2. Managing the Public Health: Incorporation or liberation?

David J Hunter

INTRODUCTION

Improving the public's health is a long-standing challenge confronting all health care systems. Health policy in most countries has it as one of its aims if not the central one. In the British NHS, the health strategy, the *Health of the Nation* in England and its equivalents elsewhere in the UK, has been concerned with achieving improved health for the population.

The 1991 NHS changes have been a catalyst to the long-running debate about how the emphasis in health policy can be shifted from health care to health. In particular, the role of health authorities as purchasers or commissioners is directed towards health improvement or health gain rather than the maintenance of the health care system which, by itself, cannot deliver on the broader health agenda. At least, it cannot do so single-handed, although it has an important contribution to make to the pursuit of health.

At the same time, concern about public health has probably never been higher with ample indications that politicians are putting the people's health at risk. While food policy and the scares over BSE and *E. coli* are at the forefront of public concern, it goes much wider. As Coote and Hunter (1996: 9) argue

People have had cause to worry about the quality and availability of water in the new era of privatised utilities, about the link between traffic density, air pollution and the rising numbers of asthma sufferers, about the impact on mental health of increasing fears about crime, about the effects of homelessness on vulnerable families and individuals, and about the links between poverty and ill-health as the income gap widens between sections of the population.

Despite successive governments having acknowledged the importance of promoting public health, the implications of doing so in a truly committed, as opposed to a symbolic, way are profound. In particular, it means not focusing simply or primarily on the treatment of illness and injury but on putting the public health agenda at the centre of policy instead of being overshadowed by the preoccupations with the NHS and a policy climate notable for its short-termism.

With contemporary health systems facing major public health challenges that are increasing in both scope and complexity, a false dichotomy has emerged between public health specialists (whether medically qualified or not) and health services management. Whereas public health specialists have generally looked outwards towards society and the health needs of the population, health service managers have tended to focus inwards on the organisation and to become captured by the pressures, and seemingly insatiable demands, of the acute sector. Notwithstanding government policy or rhetoric, it is the acute hospital sector which absorbs managers' energies and upon which their performance is judged. Such pressures are less evident in public health whose practitioners often get marginalised in the process as a result. The upshot of all this is a group of managers and a group of public health specialists who do not always share the same objectives, and who often end up working in separate compartments instead of collaboratively. Invariably, in such circumstances, public health specialists can become marginalised while managers become ever more narrowly preoccupied with a finance-driven, short-term acute sector focused agenda. The difference between these groups is neatly captured in the title of a lecture in 1987 delivered by Marc Lalonde, a former Canadian Minister for Health, 'Health Service Managers or Managers of Health?' (Evans, 1995). At present, these responsibilities are split between chief executives in the first camp and directors of public health in the other — when, that is, they are not being sucked into managing health services.

The remainder of this chapter explores the notion of public health management as a means of ameliorating, if not resolving, the tensions and dichotomies noted above. It seeks to establish whether public health management represents the means by which health policy can be rebalanced so that the pursuit of health is uppermost and better health care services are seen as a means to this end rather than, as is so often the case, being seen as an end in themselves.

WHAT IS PUBLIC HEALTH MANAGEMENT?

The concept of public health management is really quite simple (Alderslade & Hunter, 1992, 1994). It seeks to foster a shared understanding of the various pressures on managers and public health practitioners respectively through training and practice based on core concepts and a common language. The focus of public health management

is concerned with mobilising society's resources, including the specific resources of the health service sector, to improve the health of populations (Hunter, 1993: 6).

Its value lies in offering a common umbrella for the relevant groups and skills which can contribute to public health. Another way of looking at this issue, which has much in common with public health management, is to cite the notion of 'managerial epidemiology' which requires taking responsibility for health (Evans, 1995). If health care reform is about improving the health of a defined population then the primary concern of managers should not be with the health of the institution. Managerial epidemiology, in contrast, means 'the effective management of resources to maintain and promote the health of populations' (Evans *op cit*: 471). Therefore, health care managers need to understand the importance of population-based approaches to health. At the same time, public health specialists are not merely purveyors of knowledge. They are also change agents and must therefore become skilled in managing change, building coalitions of support for change, and so on.

Public health management should not be seen as concerned exclusively with the analysis of the health needs of the population, health promotion, disease prevention and the provision of primary care services. It must concern itself with the management of all resources provided from public funds intended to improve the health of the population, including acute care. Its power and strength lie in its origins, namely, the twin traditions of public health and health services management.

The objective of health improvement has a long history among public health practitioners a key group among whom — public health medicine specialists — has had twin intellectual approaches – knowledge and action – which throughout its history have gone together. Progress has resulted from a harmony of approach with sound knowledge followed by appropriate action. This concept is easy to postulate but less easy to deliver. In practice, there has been a tension between knowledge and action with many practitioners in public health focusing on knowledge rather than action. Public health management endeavours to integrate the two approaches.

The appeal of public health management, apart from its aim of linking knowledge and action, lies in its looseness and flexibility. It aims to blur the boundaries between traditional clinical epidemiology on the one hand and social epidemiology on the other. As the Chief Medical Officer for England, Dr Kenneth Calman, has observed, public health is 'an amalgamation of a series of "ologies"' (Calman, 1993). He continues:

There is no one single science and it must draw on molecular biology, clinical practice, sociology, education, politics and management science. Hence the importance of team working and of using a wide range of skills to improve health.

Calman stresses the need for links between public health and non-medical disciplines, especially when it comes to putting the findings of public health medicine into practice:

The practical implications of public health are an art and require special skills in themselves. Skills need emphasising and include both management and political skills in the communication of ideas and complex public health issues.

The concept of public health management provides an intellectual focus for collaboration between public health physicians and managers. It offers, as Evans implies, health service managers a reminder of the kind of business they are in and public health physicians an explanation of why they need to be actively involved in purchasing and not detached or passive bystanders looking on from the sidelines (Richardson *et al.*, 1994). To quote a cliché, public health management can be seen as part of the drive to make public health 'everybody's health'.

THE APPEAL OF PUBLIC HEALTH MANAGEMENT

Within the NHS, and health field more generally, public health management is gaining increasing currency. In a study of the role of public health physicians in purchasing health care (Richardson *et al.*, *op cit*), one director of public health noted:

Health authorities are moving to become public health management organisations — this is not a public health medicine takeover, but we are playing a key role in influencing the rest of the organisation. It is getting them to have a public health mind-set.

At the same time, as the study also demonstrated, managers are recognising that the concept provides an argument for getting public health physicians truly involved in the corporate endeavour. It also helps managers to recognise their own need to focus on broad issues of public health and to build public health physicians into their thinking process. As one chief executive quoted in the study by Richardson *et al.*, (*op cit*) said:

You can't be in a management role in a health authority without a strong interest in the public health agenda. The interface between the role of public health and the management process needs to be seized and eagerly embraced … . If public health wants to be involved in shaping health, don't let managers do it all by themselves and then complain later.

As Richardson *et al.*, (*op cit*: 39) argued:

Good public health input to the purchasing process should mean that public health physicians [and other practitioners of the craft] become at some points indistinguishable from other team members.

But it would be both premature and over-optimistic to claim that a wide consensus exists on the issue or that support for public health management is overwhelming. In the study already referred to, managers challenged the concept of public health management as implying too seamless a relationship between physicians who remain uneasy about their relationship to the purchasing process and who feel more comfortable confining themselves to the familiar traditional tasks and responsibilities. However, overall, managers appeared to want public health on board sitting with them at the top table shaping policy.

The management function of public health is also an intersectoral one requiring the forging of health alliances across professions and organisations, notably primary care, local government and the independent sector. Indeed, public health specialists have been charged with the task of establishing cross-boundary alliances in the pursuit of *Health of the Nation* objectives and targets.

It should not be assumed that public health management will ever be the easy option. In particular, there will always be tensions and conflicts between short-term pressures and longer term needs, ie the urgent forever driving out the important. There will always be major pressures to focus on health care service problems such as excessive demand on hospitals, bed shortages, hospital closures, long waiting-lists and waiting-times and so on. With management capacity already overstretched, it will be even more difficult to find the time and resources to develop a health gain agenda or one which truly purports to sustain the public's health (Millar, 1997). It will never be easy to measure health gain within politically sensitive (and short) timescales.

Finally, there are real questions about where a public health management function rightfully, and most logically, belongs. It is by no means axiomatic that it should reside with health authorities although for many this is clearly the most obvious and least disruptive option. But there are some practitioners and observers who believe the case for locating public health management in local government is a persuasive one and becoming more so as the NHS progressively becomes an acute service and little else. Moreover, if one studies the history of public health, its original (and some would say natural) base is in local government. Most of its achievements in the last century originated from there and many Medical Officers of Health were exemplars of a particular type and style of public health management. Of course, if the public health function were to be relocated, there might be the inevitable turf battles between environmental health officers and public health specialists but these should not be allowed to get in the way of what could be the basis for a powerful public health movement which would be less at risk of being captured by a narrow health service agenda focusing on evidence-based medicine (EBM) and clinical effectiveness. No one denies the importance of these developments, but should it fall to public health to lead on them when it puts at risk public health's core business?

Although politicians from the two main parties have rejected the local government option for health commissioning, the case for it remains an attractive one (see Harrison *et al.*, 1991; AMA, 1993; Clarke *et al.*, 1995; Cooper *et al.*, 1995). Nor has it been convincingly refuted, the case against, mounted by NAHAT, being hard to take seriously (NAHAT, 1993).

A Unifying Focus?

If the foregoing has any merit or attractions, then there is a need for public health physicians, non-medical public health specialists and managers to find an intellectual focus for joint working since each group clearly has a vital, and complementary, contribution to make. But, it is unlikely to be forthcoming if public health physicians assume territorial supremacy and take it upon themselves to be solely responsible for purchasing for health gain. This is the way of continuing interprofessional rivalry and absence of co-ordinated working. The loser will be the goal of improved health. The concept of public health management offers such a unifying focus. It is not a soft option but demands knowledge and management skills of the highest order. Public health managers must be able to adopt a strategic approach and describe and understand the health experience of populations and analyse the factors affecting health. To achieve change, skills in leadership, analytical ability and political action are essential: managers have to operate in a multi-professional, multi-agency environment and be able to achieve multi-sectoral change. Much of this work, inevitably and by definition, will require them to operate at the margins of their own organisations. To do so effectively will demand particular qualities, aptitudes and competencies (see below).

Public health managers must also place greater emphasis on health outcomes and on health promotion and disease prevention within complex political and administrative structures where most of the influences on health are beyond their direct control. Management by influence, perhaps indirectly shaping the agendas of others by getting health onto them, therefore becomes critical.

PUBLIC HEALTH MANAGEMENT IN ACTION

Coronary Heart Disease

Coronary heart disease (CHD) services can certainly be purchased within a health service system but if the population's overall health status is to be raised, then lifestyle changes and the opportunity for healthy choices must be extended within the multi-sectoral environment. Public health managers will be concerned with both elements within a comprehensive CHD programme.

Prevention of Childhood Accidents

Services for injury treatment must of course be a matter for health services but accident prevention is largely an external, multi-sectoral responsibility. The prevention of childhood injury is a classic example involving town and road planning, educationally based preventive activities, traffic calming measures and the police to mention but a few. All these groups must be drawn into a multi-sectoral alliance committed to a coherent programme for health gain. They must agree strategic targets for improving mortality and morbidity, agree operational objectives, allocate work programmes, monitor performance and review programme content and targets against performance.

SKILLS FOR PUBLIC HEALTH MANAGEMENT

Whatever else public health management may be about, being action-oriented is widely regarded as a core function. This can pose something of a culture shock to some public health specialists. As one such respondent in the study by Richardson *et al.* (*op cit*) put it

Some public health physicians are not perceived to be action- or achievement-oriented; they are perceived to be intellectually time-consuming in terms of discussions about how jolly difficult it all is.

In taking forward a multi-sectoral approach and broad-based health agenda as sketched out in the preceding section, what qualities and skills are necessary in the effective public health manager? To begin with, a number of core processes are required (Alderslade & Hunter, 1994):

- building alliances and networks with non-health service organisations; relationships will be influential rather than managerial or directive and the capacity to create and manage change leading to health improvement within this environment will be a crucial goal for organisational and personal development;
- talking and listening to the public in order better to define and respond to need;
- developing an information and intelligence database to support public health broadly defined to embrace a holistic, ecological and social perspective; this requires integrating epidemiological data with a wide range of other social science and management research;
- having a strategic framework based on health improvement, the capacity to work within alliances, knowing the views of the public;
- giving attention to the appropriate organisational form to fulfil these functions and to the development of necessary vision, culture, people and skills; in particular, it means moving away from functional departments and towards a blending of skills in task forces and project managed initiatives — such a team approach will be looser and more fluid than conventional functional departments with sometimes lengthy hierarchies.

Moving forward in respect of these processes has important implications for the requisite skills required by practitioners of public health management, regardless of their particular disciplinary backgrounds and experiences. The growing emphasis on management suggests the need for management training. However, management principles derived from conventional health bureaucracies are no longer appropriate. A criticism of management training for public health specialists has been its largely mechanistic nature (Hunter *op cit*). Curricula have remained rooted in approaches applicable to operating in a bureaucratic organisation or administrative practices and a mainly theoretical approach to management. But, the challenges posed by the new public health demand an approach to management education that emphasises the dynamic dimension of the learning organisation. What is needed are team-building skills, how to work across boundaries in flat organisations with short or non-existent hierarchies, networking skills and coping with organisational change. They are required by public health physicians alongside traditional epidemiological skills. Results are achieved through enabling, facilitating and delegating and not through top-down, command and control arrangements. Moreover, as Eskin (1992) has argued

Tolerating ambiguity, creating long-term strategies, juggling many balls in the air at once, integrating the demands of many seemingly opposing factions and at the same time working within organisational constants demands a high degree of self-esteem.

Elsewhere, Long and Eskin (1995) have suggested that public health training needs to encompass a common vision of improving health through effective change management, public advocacy and championship and working across organisation and professional boundaries. Training programmes must prepare public health professionals to function as, and to know how to be, change agents. Public health managers need to focus their efforts on changing the human environment rather than individual lifestyles.

For public health physicians, in particular, the need for management training would seem critical. Many of the subjects in the study mentioned earlier by Richardson et al. (op cit) expressed the view that they needed opportunities for experiential learning. The management training they had had gave, in the words of one, 'too much attention to knowledge and little attention to action'. Many also stressed the need, in their view, to overcome the traditional medical model with its emphasis on the individual role in decision-making. Some urged training in organisational behaviour and in understanding their particular organisational environment. Many were conscious of a need to be more politically aware, sensitive to the politics of a situation. The development of high level political skills was seen to be crucial for the survival of public health medicine. Without them 'our specialty will wither on the vine — managers will outgun us every time'. There was a strongly felt view that public health physicians could learn better how to manage conflict and to negotiate a compromise. In general, many public health physicians thought that their training might be modelled in some way on that of managers. The potential for joint training was seen to deserve exploration. Certainly, although the need to keep technical skills well honed was acknowledged, the demands of a Director of Public Health job for example were seen to require well-developed political skills.

But if roles are being blurred, which is after all the essence of public health management, then the extent to which public health training could be of benefit to non-specialists must be considered. On the management side, there are increasing calls for managers with better knowledge of public health to go alongside their managerial skills, and knowledge. In the words of one manager, from the study already referred to, managers need 'a strong interest in the public health agenda ... . You ought to be able to talk their language and to challenge them'. Managers experience many pressures on them which constitute a barrier to their adoption of a public health perspective. This is principally because, in Evans' (1995: 464) words, 'managers are expected to manage institutions, and to keep *them* healthy'. All too often, the survival and success of the organisation is an end in itself and the practice of 'managerial epidemiology', i.e. taking responsibility for health, gets neglected or ignored altogether. Evans again:

management that is focused on the health of a population might very well transfer resources away from institutions providing care services and towards other health-promoting activities outside the conventional health care system (p. 467).

So, in different ways, those contributing to, and engaged in, public health management would seek to fill any gaps in their knowledge or skill base by acquiring either relevant management skills, public health ones or a mix of the two. In this way, they would complement and enhance the skills they already possessed.

If there is a dilemma or snag in all this it is that the NHS reforms, with their reliance on competitive forces (and while these may appear rather blunt at present, or in the process of being superseded by collaborative overtures, do not be fooled by this — just wait until the changes in primary care announced towards the end of 1996, and broadly subscribed to by the Labour government, begin to grip as they will almost certainly result in a more competitive environment) to discipline provider behaviour and promote efficient care, appear to be fundamentally at odds with the notion of managerial epidemiology focused on a stable population. Not just in the UK but elsewhere, too, the appropriate mechanisms for holding managers accountable for outcomes — for the effective care of populations — remain in their infancy.

Preparing public health managers for a task that is not only exceedingly complex but also hard to attach priority to represents a major challenge for advocates of public health management. But, as was noted at the outset, with a growing sense of public unease in evidence over the state of public policy on health matters there is the prospect of a paradigm shift which could result in a radical overhaul of public health policy and practice that is long overdue (Coote & Hunter, 1996). The prospects for public health management, while not especially encouraging, are far from hopeless.

As has been established, certain competencies and qualities are critical in the effective discharge of public health management. But there has been little empirical work carried out to identify these in practice-based contexts. A small Australian study identified 'key figure' attributes for the effective public health manager as being the following:

charisma, commitment, drive, and an ability to function in a loosely regulated environment while at the same time dealing with bureaucratic processes (Lloyd, 1994: 187).

These qualities are regarded as central in attempts to foster fundamental change in the direction of health services towards measurable health gain. Developing the catalogue of competencies further, Lloyd (*op cit*: 199) reported on the need for

competencies relevant to the leadership of complex work groups — communication skills, interpersonal skills, understanding of organisational behaviour, intellect, analytic skills, planning skills, accounting skills, and an understanding of how the system works.

From the foregoing, to be truly effective public health managers require a combination of specialist technical skills and general management skills. Management training needs to be less concerned with theoretical approaches and bureaucratic organisation and focused instead on social organisation, behavioural approaches and interpersonal skills. Above all, public health training needs to be freed from the rigidities and outmoded notions associated with the dominance of the medical tradition in public health. The public health manager, who may or may not be a doctor by background, needs to be equipped with a new type of managerial focus which emphasises flexibility and interactional skills. As one regional director of public health wrote (Adam, 1992: 33)

public health practitioners should be recruited from a range of academic and working backgrounds, with training adjusted to meet individual needs. A career structure should be established for all public health practitioners — not only those from a medical background.

At the same time, public health should be a core component in the training of all those working in the NHS.

Currently there exists little appropriate training in public health management. There is much to be done to reorient training programmes to embrace the principles and competencies enunciated earlier. A Masters in Public Health Management is being offered by the Nuffield Institute for Health at the University of Leeds. A list of course contents is provided in the Annex. The course is directed towards public health specialists and managers. The training necessary for public health management requires a shift from a traditional uni-disciplinary approach to a multi-disciplinary problem-based approach.

POSSIBLE THREATS

For all their apparent enthusiasm for roles as public health managers, among those eligible for them, are many concerns, notably among public health physicians who foresee threats to their specialty from too close an association or identification with purchasing or management (Richardson *et al.*, 1994). By taking on roles which are seen to be readily interchangeable with those of others, they fear that public health physicians might come to be seen as no longer essential. If the blurring goes too far, would there be any need for a distinct public health medicine specialty at all?

It is precisely this fear of a takeover, or colonisation, by management that has led public health specialists to be wary and maintain a degree of independence from the corporate agenda. It may be thought that public health management means the incorporation of public health and its displacement from promoting the public's health. But, it can equally be viewed as a form of liberation, enabling public health to lead and influence change towards improving the population's health. In addition, it has to be acknowledged that a potential threat exists to what some might regard as the most valuable contribution of public health which is to serve as the professional conscience of the organisation and the guardian of the public's health. Undoubtedly, there has to be a trade-off between maintaining such purist detachment, on the one hand, and being able to effect real change on the other.

Public health management requires all those with an interest or skill in public health to seize the corporate agenda and make it central to the mission and core business of the authority. That public health medicine, as a key component of public health management, feels insecure and lacking in confidence is evident from Salter's (1993: 28) diagnosis of the specialty's malaise following the 1991 NHS reforms:

Public health medicine does not have unique control over, and access to, a particular body of knowledge — the characteristic possessed by all powerful professional groups. Over recent years it has expanded its concerns to include not only the causal antecedents of a new set of diseases associated

with inequalities in health, demographic shifts, industrialisation and ecological imbalance but also the interagency policies required to deal with
these issues …. It has stretched itself too thinly and too far.

All the more reason, then, for public health physicians and others
involved in the specialty of public health medicine to embrace public
health management. Within the developing purchasing environment,
the need for the combined expertise of many different professionals is
not in dispute. The agenda cannot be the sole preserve of any particular body of expertise — it is simply too big and multi-faceted. It can
only be tackled effectively by a multi-skilled and managed approach.
This should both reassure and enthuse all those with an interest in
promoting the public's health from a public health perspective.

While all of these arguments are persuasive and make intuitive
sense, there are also risks which need to be acknowledged in order
to do something to remove them or reduce their impact. Health policy is riven with paradoxes. Charles Handy (1994) argues that paradox is a fact of life — it is 'inevitable, endemic and perpetual'.
Paradox is a consequence of complexity and turbulence. The trick
is to manage it because, like the weather, it has to be lived with, not
resolved. Many paradoxes and contradictions face those who are
obvious candidates for public health management roles and responsibilities. For example:

- we talk continually of health but our focus remains firmly on
  ill-health and disease – as has often been remarked, we do not
  have a *health* service but a *sickness* service;
- public health as it has evolved in the NHS over the past 20
  years or so has become captured by ever narrower health service
  issues and interests and is in danger of losing sight of its true
  public health ethos;
- for all the talk of the health of local populations and of health
  needs assessment, the focus of policy makers is firmly on hospital services, acute care, beds, waiting lists and 'bricks and mor-
  tar' issues; such biases are a product of the notorious efficiency
  index but also of the mindset of those operating within the
  NHS who for the most part come from a tradition of providing
  care rather than providing or supporting health;
- while the rhetoric stresses collaboration and partnership, the
  reality, partly as a consequence of various reforms in public
  services whether in health, education or community care, is
  increasingly about growing fragmentation and pluralism with
  competing interests a feature of health policy;

- fragmentation and competitive principles have substituted low trust relations for high trust ones;
- instead of embracing complexity, problems are disaggregated into single issues and discrete, manageable chunks with the result that highly complex issues, which in reality are interdependent, are oversimplified – the analogy might be moving from shining a spotlight on a particular problem to throwing a lighthouse beam across the whole area of a particular policy field.

Rather than be engulfed by these paradoxes, which of course must always be a danger, public health management may represent the means whereby they can be more effectively managed.

THE END OF INNOCENCE: A CONCLUDING COMMENT

It is sometimes suggested that public health specialists are 'dreamers' while, in contrast, managers are 'pragmatists' (Richardson *et al.*, *op cit*). They are the 'doers', while public health specialists dream up unworkable schemes and comment on how difficult it all is. But, this polarisation is false and a growing appreciation exists of the need for a synthesis between the two perspectives. Public health management provides such a synthesis.

Arguably, public health as a field of inquiry, with public health medicine as a major specialty contributing to it together with those working in public health and related areas but who are not medically qualified, is gaining in importance. As was stressed at the outset, the issue of, and interest in, public health have never been more important. That more and more skills should become part of public health is a welcome development. The term 'public health management' provides an umbrella for all these while also seeking to clarify and give a sharper focus to the public health challenge and to the means of meeting it. This can be no bad thing when those working in public health complain of being stretched too thinly across a whole range of functions which often appear peripheral to their core business. Such a state of affairs certainly serves to dissipate their efforts and weakens any impact they might otherwise have.

But while the purchasing task may provide that focus and discipline in terms of what public health should concentrate on, it is just conceivable that public health is being offered a poisoned chalice (Richardson *et al.*, 1994). Public health may be central to the purchasing task but if the expectations of it are not met and public health fails to deliver then it will almost certainly suffer a severe setback from which it may not recover (Richardson *et al.*, *op cit*: 44).

As health authorities engage in the intricacies of maintaining an acceptable balance of health care while attempting to nudge services towards the achievement of more strategic goals,

those involved in public health may find themselves carrying an impossible or unacceptable burden. Failure to deliver on the public health agenda could bring in its wake a search for scapegoats. Public health physicians are vulnerable in such circumstances as history has shown (Lewis, 1986). But, this surely strengthens the case for public health management if seen as an endeavour for which many skills are needed and for which no one discipline or group can claim all credit if things go well or be blamed if they do not. In short, public health management must become the means of implementing the corporate agenda and, in the process, of becoming inseparable from it.

Growing pressures to deliver cost-effective health care could, however unlikely it seems from the present standpoint, finally persuade politicians that public health management is a valuable tool to provide the seamless linkage between prevention, promotion, primary care and acute services as well as between the NHS and all those other agencies whose activities impact so crucially on health. The appointment of the first ever minister of Public Health and the announcement of a new, broad-based health strategy to be launched in July 1998 are moves in the right direction.

REFERENCES

Adam S 1992 What business is public health medicine in? Personal views. Journal of Management in Medicine 6: 32–4
Alderslade R, Hunter D J 1992 Forward March. Health Service Journal 102: 22–3
Alderslade R, Hunter D J 1994 Commissioning and public health. Journal of Management in Medicine 8: 20–31
Association of Metropolitan Authorities 1993 Local Authorities and Health Services: A future role for local authorities in the purchasing of health services. A Scoping Paper. AMA, London
Calman K 1993 The Scientific Basis of Public Health. Address to the Annual Conference of the Faculty of Public Health Medicine. Glasgow
Clarke M, Hunter D J, Wistow G 1995 Local Government and the NHS: The new agenda. Local Government Management Board, Luton
Cooper L, Coote A, Davis A et al 1995 Voices Off: Tackling the democratic deficit in health. Institute for Public Policy Research, London
Coote A, Hunter D J 1996 New Agenda for Health. Institute for Public Policy Research, London
Eskin F 1992 Sex, violence and public health physicians. Public Health Physician 3
Evans R G 1995 Healthy populations or healthy institutions: the dilemma of health care management. The Journal of Health Administration Education 13: 453–72
Handy C 1994 The Empty Raincoat. Hutchinson, London
Harrison S, Hunter D J, Johnston I et al 1991 Health Before Health Care. Institute for Public Policy Research, London

Hunter D J 1993 Public health management: implications for training. HFA 2000 News 23: 5–7

Lewis J 1986 What Price Community Medicine? The Philosophy, Practice and Politics of Public Health Since 1919. Wheatsheaf Books, Brighton

Lloyd P 1994 Management competencies in health for all/new public health settings. The Journal of Health Administration Education 12: 187–207

Long A F, Eskin F 1995 The new public health: changing attitudes and practice. Medical Principles and Practice 4: 171–8

Millar B 1997 Nine-to-five. Health Service Journal 107: 12–13

National Association of Health Authorities and Trusts 1993 Securing Effective Public Accountability in the NHS: A discussion paper. NAHAT, Birmingham

Richardson A, Duggan M, Hunter D J 1994 Adapting to New Tasks: The role of public health physicians in purchasing health care. Nuffield Institute for Health, Leeds

Salter B 1993 Public image limited. Health Service Journal 103: 28

APPENDIX

MA IN PUBLIC HEALTH MANAGEMENT

Course content

Core module

- Foundations of public health management.

Elective modules

- Strategic management;
- Finance, budgets and markets in health and social care;
- Economics of health and social care;
- Health and social care policy;
- Basic epidemiology and statistics;
- Population based research;
- Assessing effectiveness and outcomes.

Optional modules

- Medical sociology;
- Ethical issues in health and social care;
- Marketing for health and social care;
- Assessing organisational performance;
- Primary and community care;
- Theories and models of quality assurance;
- Health care in an international perspective.

Assessment

Applications

3. Health for All: The new millennium

John Ashton

THE STRATEGY OF HEALTH FOR ALL BY THE YEAR 2000

The Strategy of Health for All by the year 2000 was adopted as policy by the World Health Assembly in 1981 building on the acceptance by the 1977 Assembly...'that the main social target of governments and of the WHO should be the attainment by all the people of the world by the year 2000 of a level of health that will permit them to lead a socially and economically productive life... ' and on the declaration that emerged from the WHO and UNICEF sponsored conference the following year in Alma-Ata in the former USSR which stated that primary health care is the key to attaining this target (WHO, 1981).This high-falluting and millennial-sounding objective has been much criticised as mere rhetoric by overpaid international bureaucrats as indeed much of the work of the WHO itself has been criticised . However, the Health for All initiative did not occur in a vacuum, even if its conception owed much to the vision and energy of the WHO's charismatic Director General, Dr Halfdan Mahler. Rather, it was the manifestation of a debate about the mission of medicine and the task of public health which had begun to move from the academic to the practical (Kickbusch, 1986; Ashton & Seymour 1988). The outcome to date has in fact been far more practical than some of Health for All's esoteric critics from academia would allow, as many governments have embarked on the arduous task of reorienting their health systems with all that entails in terms of confronting vested and entrenched interests in the professions, in education and research establishments and among the providers of public services. When history is written, I would expect that the progress which has been made to date with Mahler's 'healthy virus', as he is said to have described the necessary process to achieve the goal of Health for All to be given more credit than its detractors would allow just 20 years after the Alma Ata meeting.

WHY HEALTH FOR ALL WAS NECESSARY

I have discussed elsewhere the three phases that can be identified in public health in the developed world during the past 150 years (Ashton & Seymour, 1988).The environmental and sanitary emphasis of the early period (c 1840–1880) would not have seemed strange to Hippocrates himself who wrote in his treatise that

whoever would apply himself right to physick should observe this method. First, he should consider the Seasons of the year, and what every one is capable of producing: for they are not at all alike, but differ much from one another, and in their several changes. Secondly, the Winds, both the hot and the cold, especially those that are common to all Nations; and, next to these, such as are peculiar to certain Countries. Thirdly, the Waters, and their several qualities: for as they differ in taste and weight, so the virtue of every one differs considerably. For which reason when a man comes a perfect stranger to a City, he should consider well the situation of it, how it stands with respect to the Winds, and the risings of the Sun... (Francis Clifton, MD 1734)

Similarly the growth of personal prevention measures in the later part of the 19th century with the advent of immunisation, of family planning and school and community-based preventive initiatives including the provision of school meals in some countries would probably have made sense to the followers of the Greek Goddess, Hygieia, for whom health was the natural order of things, a positive attribute to which people were entitled if they led their lives wisely (McKeown, 1976). Similarly the tension between the Hygieians and the Asclepians, more sceptical in their belief that, whilst discovering and teaching the natural laws which would ensure a healthy mind in a healthy body was all very well, in the real world the role of the physician was to treat disease and to restore health by correcting any imperfections caused by the accidents of birth and life has its echoes in the conflict which has often seemed to exist between prevention and therapy since therapeutics moved into the ascendancy in the 1930s and 1940s.The debate which ushered in the fourth phase, which has come to be known as the New Public Health and to which the Health for All strategy belongs, has its origins in a number of strands of critique and in the dawning realisation that, whilst a healthy tension between different emphases in health and health care might be one thing, the wholesale eclipsing of one perspective by another was altogether different and it risked not only the negligent abandonment of 150 years of experience and expertise but was also a threat to the public health in its own right. This debate can be traced to a growing awareness of the limitations of scientific medicine. McKeown's widely quoted Rock Carling lecture of 1976 in which he argued that:

in order of importance the major contributions to improvements in health in England and Wales were from limitations of family size (a behavioural change, increase in food supplies and a healthier physical environment (environmental influences) and specific preventive and therapeutic measures. McKeown, 1976)

Illich's strident critique of modern medicine is itself a kind of epidemic and a major cause of 'disease' (Illich, 1975) and the growing body of literature on inequalities in health which seemed to indicate that if anything modern medicine was serving to increase the health gap between the advantaged and disadvantaged, (for example, Tudor Hart, 1971; Townsend, 1974), all contributed to the momentum as too did the international financial crises of the early 1970s which served to throw the spotlight on the escalating costs of medical care and raised questions about their commensurate benefits. The coalescence of concern and the emergence of a revitalised concept of primary care such as to ground it in a population and environment or public health perspective (Box 3.1) had much to do with growing international disillusionment with the failure of the fashionably marketed concepts of acute general and university hospitals and highly trained groups of scientific health professionals to do other than pander to the needs of ruling elites. The bringing of the new thinking together in a practical way for the first time fell to the Canadian minister of health Lalonde who published *A New Perspective On The Health Of Canadians* in 1974, a report which was to prove influential globally as a model for community diagnoses and intelligence-based health policy and feeding into the thinking which led to the Alma Ata conference in 1977 (Lalonde, 1974). Waiting in the wings, as it were, for the moment was the Rock Carling lecture of 1971 by Archie Cochrane on the theme of Effectiveness and Efficiency, subtitled 'Random Reflections on Health Services' in which he developed his thesis on what we would 20 years later come to term 'Evidence-based Health Care' (Cochrane, 1972).

It seems ironic now that the period of greatest public investment in medical care that preceded the belt-tightening of the 1970s should have missed the opportunity of building on a consensus understanding of the task which had prevailed until after the end of

Box 3.1 The eight elements of primary health care

1. Health education;
2. Food supply and proper nutrition;
3. Safe water and basic sanitation;
4. Maternal and child health care;
5. Immunisation;
6. Prevention and control of endemic diseases;
7. Basic treatment of health problems;
8. Provision of essential drugs.

Source: Vuori, H. (1984).

the second world war. In 1941, Sigerist was articulating a commonly held view when he wrote his 'Outline Health programme for Every Country' as including:

- free education for all the people including health education;
- the best possible working and living conditions;
- the best possible means of rest and recreation;
- a system of health institutions and medical personnel available to all;
- centres of medical training and research.

Yet, within a short time, much of this holistic thinking began to be lost under the onslaught of reductionist quick-fixes and it would be more than 20 years before Winslow's 1920s definition of Public Health would again command proper attention

Public Health is the science and art of preventing disease, prolonging life and promoting physical health and efficiency through organised community efforts for the sanitation of the environment, the education of the individual in principles of personal hygiene, the organisation of medical and nursing service for the early diagnosis and preventive treatment of disease, and the development of the social machinery which will ensure to every individual in the community a standard of living adequate for the maintenance of health (Winslow, 1920)

THE CHANGING TASK OF PUBLIC HEALTH

So far, this account of the changing shape and emphasis of public health responses has made little reference to the changing task confronting its practitioners. In developed countries, for example, there have been dramatic changes in the demographic structure, in the patterns of health and disease and in the capacity of interventions whether technical or social to make a difference. By way of illustration, a report on the changing health of the Mersey Region of England between 1948 and 1994 makes quite vivid reading (Ashton, 1995). At the outset of the period in a Region of over 2 million people, there were some 40,000 births annually; by 1994, there were only just over 30,000. Whereas in 1948 childbearing commonly began in the teens or early 20s with families of four and more children being commonplace, by the 1990s it had become the norm to defer childbearing to the late 20s and for women, on average, to have less than two children. In 1948, 50 out of every 1000 children born would not live to see their first birthday and many of them were still carried off by infectious diseases as indeed were their parents. Fifty years later, this toll had been reduced to 7, of which perhaps two-thirds were attributable to genetic causes at present not amenable to prevention. At the other end of the age scale, men were now living on average into their 70s and women were commonly reaching 80 or more, despite a regional concentration of adverse living and working conditions. Overall, a population structure with less than 5% pensioners at the turn of the century now had approaching 20%, and one of the fastest growing groups was the over-85s of whom perhaps one-third will be suffering from brain failure. The implications which follow from this demographic change are that chronic non-communicable and degenerative diseases requiring locally based high quality continuing care have largely replaced infectious disease as the major public health challenges of the second half of the century together with a growing recognition of the importance of mental health.

The third leg of the tripod of needs assessment is the capacity of interventions to make a difference, together with public perceptions and expectations of what services they require; frustratingly, for many health professionals, the evidence-based approach to the provision of public services, assuming as it does a rational approach to life in general is frequently at odds with the way in which all of us actually live. Nevertheless, whereas McKeown could argue that, until the 1920s, there were precious few effective medical or surgical treatments, the post-war period has been characterised by an explosion of therapeutic possibilities, both pharmacological and otherwise. Changes in approach, such as the massive increase in day surgery made possible by a combination of changed surgical techniques, new anaesthetic agents and changed public expectations, have dramatically changed the characteristics of hospital work. It is possible too that the very efficacy of many modern treatments is, itself, part of the explanation of the renewed interest in community-based practice, for when hospital is no longer the referral point of last resort but actually has something to offer, why should that expertise not be disseminated among community-based practitioners in the same way that other technologies, having been developed in specialist centres, are rolled out and made available on a large scale and at lower unit costs?

These three factors: changed demography, changed epidemiology and changed possibilities and expectations have transformed and are transforming the task facing public health. They are factors which have been reinforced by a further set of major trends, which include the spread of universal education and the rapid growth in further and higher education and information technology, which serve to undermine the traditional preciousness of professional groups and the protection of their position of authority based on control of the knowledge base; a growing awareness of the ecological dimensions of health among the general public assisted by the mass media, even if such an awareness has so far made little inroad into the institutions training health care professionals; a similar general trend towards multi-disciplinary and multi-professional ways of working (yet to be properly supported by a re-orientation of training institutions), and the globalisation of life in general and of the public health agenda in particular (drugs, HIV/AIDS, plague, cholera, acid rain, global warming, terrorism and man-made disasters such as Chernobyl, heart disease, cancer, teenage pregnancy and road traffic accidents and car-generated atmospheric pollution).

METHODS, ACHIEVEMENTS AND EXPERIENCES

In my opinion, there can be little doubt that one of the major achievements of the past 20 years has been the emergence of a coherent approach to promoting and protecting the health of the population, in particular as articulated in the Ottawa Charter for Health Promotion. Five key principles lie behind the charter in its emphasis on policies to support health, the creation of supportive environments, strengthening community action, developing personal skills and reorientating health services.

1. Heath promotion actively involves the population in the setting of everyday life rather than focusing on people who are at risk for specific conditions and in contact with medical services.

2. Health promotion is directed at action on the causes of ill-health.
3. Health promotion uses many different approaches which combine to improve health. These include education and information, community development and organisation, health advocacy and legislation.
4. Health promotion depends particularly on public participation.
5. Health professionals—especially those in primary care—have an important part to play in nurturing health promotion and enabling it to take place (WHO *et al.*, 1986).

This final point is particularly important in that it implies that one of the major changes which is needed is in the working ethos and style of a whole range of heath professionals and in the policy emphasis of a wide range of public, private and voluntary sector organisations. Contrary to occasional rumour, the main purpose of health promotion is not the creation of a new professional group or to provide jobs for people running new courses. Reorientation of existing policies, practices, and professionals is both critical and central. (Nor is heath promotion a specific agenda confined to the so-called lifestyle issues: drugs/alcohol/tobacco/sex/obesity/exercise, etc, which sometimes seems to be a way of recycling health education officers without fundamentally changing anything.)

The Ottawa Charter has been influential in giving shape to a wide range of seemingly disparate activities and initiatives. It is difficult to overstate how important this is. In the post-modern context of multiple social groups where the emphasis is on diversity and voluntarism rather than on homogeneity and coercion and automatic legislation, one of the real dangers is that there will be growing inequities in health which reflect the differing inherent strengths of different neighbourhoods, localities and communities. In this situation the challenge is to develop a strategic approach which can underpin the diversity and facilitate differing populations going forward at a similar pace. One such strategic approach has been the WHO sponsored Healthy City Initiative (Ashton *et al.*, 1986; Ashton, 1992). The intention behind this initiative was to try and take the approach which came to underpin the Ottawa Charter and to apply it at a level where there were mechanisms of governance in place such as to support the development and implementation of appropriate health promoting policies in a very practical way. The initiative was, in fact, drawing on the real and effective experiences which came from the Victorian public health movement in England in the 1840s when the Health of Towns Association achieved a significant measure of success in obtaining sanitary reform through a combination of intelligence gathering, lobbying and advocacy and community organisation (Ashton & Ubido,1991).The Heathy Cities Project proposed a city level agenda for action based on joint working of the Health and Local Authorities and the voluntary sector with further partnerships which included academics, the business community and the media. Some 10 years on, it is possible to reflect on the experience of an initiative which has genuinely been taken up globally. On the positive side the initiative has raised the profile of urban health in a very significant way and at its best has enabled organisations which have historically been in conflict to develop joint strategies; on the negative side, there are many examples of what can only be described as 'projectism', where there has been no impact in terms of fundamental reorientation of policy and practice but rather Healthy Cities (or towns and communities) has remained a series of disconnected and often sidelined projects. Often connected to this failure has been what could only be described as either a failure of vision and strategic thinking or perhaps more frequently a reluctance by a particular professional or other occupational or interest group to pursue the intended goal of a win–win situation rather than the pursuit of personal or craft self-interest. (WHO, 1993; Liverpool City Health Plan 1996)

LOOKING AHEAD BEYOND THE MILLENNIUM

The millennium is upon us and we don't have Health for All. What we do have is a rapid and growing pace of change where a shrinking world looks forward to a stabilising global population in the second half of the century and the progressive blurring of what are first and what are third world health problems. On recent experience, there is the emergence of threats to health from the environment, from lifestyles and behaviours and from the other organisms with which we share the planet. Impressionistically, it seems that, if the 1980s was the decade in which there was a reawakening of awareness about personal prevention, the 1990s has seen a progressive sensitisation to environmental questions. As telecommunications and jet travel accelerate the realisation of Mcluhan's prediction of the global village, it remains to be seen whether this sensitisation can be translated into consensual policy and effective action rapidly enough to prevent the inevitable threats to public health from the degradation of the environment and pressure on natural eco-systems from approaching 10 billion people wishing to behave in the same way as Northern Europeans, the North Americans or increasing numbers of residents of the Pacific rim. One thing is certain and that is that a professionalocentric approach to health, whereby the public is expected to relinquish the ownership of the health agenda to experts of whatever hue, is not only unlikely to meet the needs of the times but is likely to be by-passed by events. However, professionals and other interest groups cannot be expected to stand by passively while populism undermines their power base; indeed, there are already signs of regrouping going on around the clinical effectiveness agenda, for example. This agenda can be construed as seeking to create a new sect of meta-reductionist priests or gurus presiding over the randomised, controlled trial as the contemporary version of the magic bullet — an equally unsophisticated tool for understanding people's existential dilemmas of being and experiencing health and disease in the world. Threatening, too, to the assumption that on the coat-tails of global telecommunications must follow an empowered and participating global citizenry is the concentration of wealth into fewer and fewer global corporate hands and the alternative nightmare scenario as described in David Korten's book *When Corporations Rule the World* raises the prospect of a new era of global feudalism, wherein the majority of the world's population is to be found in a sophisticated type of new serfdom (Korten, 1995). No shortage of challenges for the New Public Health in the new millennium then!

REFERENCES

Ashton J, Grey P, Barnard K 1986 Healthy Cities: WHO's New Public Health Initiative. Health Promotion 1(3): 319–23
Ashton J, Seymour H 1988 The New Public Health. Open University Press
Ashton J, Ubido J 1991 The healthy city and the ecological idea.The Society for the Social History of Medicine 14(1): 173–81
Ashton J (ed) 1992 Healthy Cities. Open University Press
Ashton J 1995 The Changing Health of Mersey 1948–1994. Report of the Mersey Regional Director of Public Health. Mersey R.H.A. Liverpool
Cochrane A 1972 Effectiveness and Efficiency. Random Reflections on Health Services. Nuffield Provincial Hospitals Trust
Illich I 1975 Medical Nemesis — The Expropriation of Health.
Kickbusch I 1986 Health promotion. Strategies for action. Canadian Journal of Public Health 77(5): 321–6
Korten D 1995 When Corporations Rule the World. Kumarian Press and Berrett-Koehler
Lalonde M 1974 A New Perspective on the Health of Canadians. Minister of Supply and Services
Liverpool Health Authority 1996 The City Health Plan
McKeown T 1976 The Role of Medicine — Dream, mirage or nemesis. Nuffield Provincial Hospitals Trust

Miller J 1971 McLuhan. Fontana/Collins
Sigerist H 1941 Medicine and Human Welfare. Oxford University Press
Townsend P 1974 Inequality and the Health Service. Lancet i: 1179–90
Tudor-Hart J 1971 The inverse care law. Lancet i: 405–12
Vuori H 1984 Primary health care in Europe: problems and solutions. Community
     Health 6: 221–31
WHO 1981 Global Strategy for Health for All by the Year 2000.WHO, Geneva
WHO, Health and Human Welfare Canada, Canadian Public Health Association
     1986 Ottawa Charter for Health Promotion.WHO, Copenhagen
WHO 1993 The Urban Health Crisis. WHO, Geneva
Winslow CEA 1920 The untilled fields of public health. Science 51: 23

4. Public Health and European Integration

Martin McKee and Elias Mossialos

INTRODUCTION

Anyone who thought that public health practitioners could ignore the consequences of European integration must surely have had their views dispelled by the introduction in 1996 by the European Commission of a world-wide ban on the export of British beef, on grounds of public health. This has had enormous political and financial consequences for the United Kingdom, leading to the loss of thousands of jobs and millions of pounds in export revenue as well as a period of non-co-operation with our European partners that has caused severe damage to Britain's reputation (McKee *et al.*, 1996a).

This is, however, only the most visible example of how Europe is influencing public health practice in the United Kingdom. The process of European integration has many consequences for public health practitioners and researchers, some obvious and others less so. This chapter seeks to identify some of them. It begins with a brief description of the relevant European institutions. It continues with a discussion of some of the ways that the growing volume of European law is affecting public health and a description of official European policies on public health and health-related research. It concludes with an exploration of the opportunities offered by closer union for learning from experience elsewhere.

THE STRUCTURES OF THE EUROPEAN UNION

The objective of ever closer union, established in the Treaty of Rome and developed through successive European treaties, most recently that signed at Amsterdam, has led to the creation of a European tier of government, with executive, legislative and judicial functions. It makes laws that are the basis of policies which it implements, and enforces those laws through court judgements. The following paragraphs summarise how this process works.

The four main bodies involved are the Commission, the Council of Ministers, the European Parliament, and the European Court of Justice, although there are also other bodies that may have a role in certain circumstances. The responsibility for initiating legislation lies with the Commission. This is a body of 20 Commissioners, one appointed by each member state except the UK, Germany, France, Italy and Spain, each of whom appoint two. It is headed by a president from among this number. Formally, once appointed, the Commissioners are independent of their national governments who may not sack them but can refuse to renew their appointments. As at national level, legislation emerges from a process of consultation with interest groups, national experts, and senior civil servants. It is also possible for the Council (see below) to ask the Commission to undertake studies and submit proposals. Proposals for new treaties generally emerge from the Council. The initiation and progress of a proposal is often the responsibility of a single commissioner, but he or she must retain the support of a majority of the Commission to ensure its survival. Decisions are taken on a simple majority, and there is collective responsibility.

Once agreed, a proposal is presented to the Council of Ministers. This is the body responsible, in most cases, for agreeing the content of European law. It consists of a general council (attended by foreign ministers) and a series of specialist councils (such as health) attended by the relevant ministers. The presidency of the council rotates on a six-monthly basis among the member states and, as the president controls the agenda, this provides an opportunity for national governments to influence the direction in which the Union is moving. A disadvantage is that a country's presidency may coincide with a period of domestic political turmoil or even a general election, reducing the overall effectiveness of the council. To add to the complication, it is important to note the separate existence of the 'European Council'. This meets twice a year, often attracting considerable media interest, and is attended by heads of government. It does not have the power to make laws but does provide a general direction for the development of the Union.

The Council of Ministers adopts legislation by voting. There are a few situations, largely to do with procedural matters, in which a simple majority is sufficient. In practice, however, most laws are subject to either unanimity or qualified majority votes. The former is self-explanatory. The latter is a system whereby each country's votes are weighted to reflect differences in population size. Out of a possible 87, 62 votes are needed to pass legislation. In practice, this means that at least three states, including two of the larger ones, can block it. This has been the situation with, for example, the proposed ban on tobacco advertising which was opposed by the UK, Germany, Netherlands and Denmark (Chapman, 1991). A change of policy under the new British government will thus have Europe-wide consequences. A point worth reiterating is that, despite a tendency in the UK to blame 'Brussels' for unpopular legislation, that legislation can only come about if our ministers either approve it or, in some circumstances, fail to persuade sufficient others of their arguments. Furthermore, those situations in which European law has been enacted, which clearly fails to take into account the circumstances of the UK, such as a directive requiring that abattoirs must have a vet (who in many continental countries is the equivalent of a meat inspector but is a rather more expensive veterinary surgeon in the UK) are often due to a failure of government to scrutinise draft legislation adequately, a failure not limited to European legislation (Marr, 1995).

The third major body is the European Parliament. It has been directly elected since 1979 and is similar in size to the House of Commons, with 626 members. Members sit according to multi-national political groups, of which the largest, with 221 members, is currently the Party of European Socialists, which includes the British Labour Party. In addition to its plenary meetings, much work takes place in committees, such as that responsible for environment, health and consumer protection. The principal role of the parliament has been to supervise the other community institutions and, especially the Commission. It does so through questions and publication of reports, rather like the way in which a British parliamentary select committee works.

In the area of legislation, it may be involved through a process of consultation or co-operation. The process to be used in a particular case is set out in the relevant articles of the treaties. In the former case, the Council of Ministers must ask parliament for an opinion on proposed legislation. It is not permitted to vote on it until it has received that opinion so, although the views of parliament can be ignored, it can impose severe delays if amendments are not accepted. The second process, which has expanded greatly, is co-operation, in which, following consultation, the Council of Ministers adopts a common position that is referred back to parliament for a second reading. Parliament can then amend or reject the legislation when, for the unammended version to pass into law, it must be agreed by the Council of Ministers by unanimity. For example, the view of the Commission and Council that cars under 1.4 litres capacity should not require catalytic converters was rejected by the parliament and the Council was unable to overturn this. Finally, the Maastricht Treaty gave parliament the power of veto, subject to a conciliation procedure, in limited areas but including incentive measures related to public health. For completeness, it should be noted that there are two other bodies that must be consulted about legislation in some areas. These are the Committee of the Regions (consisting of nominees of local government) and the Economic and Social Committee (representing industry and trade unions). Neither committee can, however, impose delays or block legislation, and thus they are seen as relatively powerless. The latter is, however, credited by some with identifying inconsistencies in proposed legislation.

The fourth major body is the European Court of Justice. It consists of 15 judges and nine advocate-generals, appointed by common accord of the member states for a renewable term of six years. Those appointed are normally already senior judges in their own countries but can include senior academic lawyers. Advocates-general do not correspond with a British position and their role is derived from French jurisprudence. They are responsible for summarising the case for the judges, including the preparation of a comprehensive review of relevant European law, and giving an opinion, which is not binding on the judges, on how the court should decide the case. As will be seen later, the Court is taking an increasingly important role in the evolution of European law.

The process of lawmaking at a European level continues to evolve. One of the major forces behind current changes is expansion of the Union. Following the most recent expansion there has been greater pressure for transparency of decision-making in the Council of Ministers, largely in response to Swedish concerns. The increasing size of the Union has, itself, certain consequences. It is now recognised by most member states that the retention of a national veto in many areas brings the risk of paralysis of decision-making. It is fine whenever it is oneself using the veto but less satisfactory when an important national objective is blocked by another country pursuing a narrow domestic agenda. Finally, in each of the successive treaties, the power of the European Parliament has been increasing. Many see this as essential if the institutions of the

European Union are to attract wider popular support. Of course, a stronger parliament can become a threat to national politicians, even if it is good for democracy as a whole.

THE EFFECT OF EUROPEAN LAW AT NATIONAL LEVEL

The concept of parliamentary sovereignty, as enshrined in the 1688 Bill of Rights, has been an article of faith in the United Kingdom In a wider European context, this freedom, which in practice resides with the executive due to the tight control of British parliamentary parties (Jenkins, 1995), is an anachronism. Most other governments accept that their freedom of action is constrained by a constitution, frequently backed by a constitutional court. In practice, however, the activities of the British government are constrained by various international treaties, the most important of which are those relating to accession to the European Community and the subsequent development of our relationship with what is now the European Union. In particular, the 1972 European Communities Act, which provided the legal basis for our accession to the Community, in section 2(I) gave the force of law in the United Kingdom to those provisions of Community law that have direct effect regardless of whether they were enacted before or subsequent to our accession. Exactly which elements of Community law have 'direct effect' is too complex an issue to explore here (Weatherill & Beaumont, 1996) but, for the present purposes, the key issue is that section 3(I) of the Act required the British government to accept the judgement of the European Court of Justice on which provisions of Community law have this effect. This situation has steadily evolved through rulings of the European Court and House of Lords which, to simplify a complicated situation, can be summarised as establishing the principle of supremacy of European law over national law and introducing the principle that national law enacted to implement community directives should be consistent with the purpose the directive seeks to achieve rather than a narrow technical interpretation of its wording. Consequently, contrary to what some politicians might wish, parliament has quite explicitly constrained its own sovereignty and, by virtue of the process of qualified majority voting, is required to give force of law to various policies which it might disagree with. Thus, as is increasingly apparent in, for example, the ban on export of British beef and the consequences for contracting out of ancillary services in the National Health

Service of the Transfer of Undertakings (Protection of Employment) directive, European law is destined to play an increasingly important part in the evolution of national policies on a wide range of issues. In the present context, it is the impact of European law on public health that is of interest. This chapter cannot possibly deal with this topic exhaustively and a more detailed review of its impact on national health policy has recently been published elsewhere (McKee et al., 1996b). Instead, this chapter will focus on those areas of most direct importance for public health practice and policies. Before doing so, however, it is necessary briefly to summarise the different components of European law. The first of these consist of the various treaties, including those signed at Rome and Maastricht. As noted above, an individual can seek redress in the British courts to have these treaties enforced, both as they apply to a dispute between him or her and the government (vertical effect) or with another individual (horizontal effect). As noted above, the treaties give the European Union competence to enact regulations and directives in various areas, through a process in which, most commonly, they are proposed by the Commission and agreed by the Council of Ministers (representing national governments) and the European Parliament. Regulations have direct effect in member states but directives set out objectives that national governments must then enact legislation to achieve, taking into account national circumstances, but bearing in mind the emphasis on the purpose of the directive, as noted above. Directives must be enacted nationally within a defined period and, if a member state fails to do so, an individual may seek redress in a national court on the basis of the directive, leading to a situation in which a directive may pass into national law in a way in which parliament may not have intended. While all of these instruments set out the general direction of European law, in practice, as with national law, it is the responsibility of the courts to determine the detailed applicability in a particular case. Although the European Court is not bound by its own earlier decisions, it does commonly follow them, thus establishing through precedent an evolving body of law which, in practice, can lead to consequences not always foreseen when the corresponding treaties, regulations and directives were agreed. This often arises as the Court will interpret law in a contextual and purposive manner, having regard for the treaty provisions and, in particular, the agreement of member states to move towards ever closer union.

The extent to which the European Union has specific competence in the field of public health is relatively limited. The 1957
Treaty of Rome, while establishing the 'four freedoms' of movement
of goods, persons, services, and capital, in Article 36 empowered
member states to limit movement of goods on grounds of protection
of human health and life. The Treaty, and the earlier treaties establishing Euratom and the European Coal and Steel Community, also
contained some provisions relating to health and safety at work.
The 1985 Single European Act introduced the requirement for the
Community to make a high level of health protection the basis for
its proposals in the field of health, safety, and environmental and
health protection. However the most important change came with
the 1991 Maastricht Treaty which, in Article 129, gave the
Community specific competence in public health, enabling it to
adopt incentive measures to encourage member states to address
prevention of diseases and ensure that health protection shall be a
part of the Community's other policies. The specific actions undertaken to achieve these objections will be discussed later. In the next
section, some of the ways in which the 'four freedoms' that are the
basic principles of European law can influence public health policies and practice will be considered.

IMPLICATIONS FOR POSTGRADUATE MEDICAL TRAINING

The right of health professionals to practise in another member
state was established in the Treaty of Rome. The detailed arrangements have subsequently been set out in a series of directives relating to doctors, dentists, pharmacists, nurses and midwives. In brief,
these abolish restrictions based on the national origin of qualifications and enable suitably qualified staff the right to practise elsewhere after application to a designated responsible authority in the
host country. The general principle underlying these policies is that
of mutual recognition which means that, providing a country's
qualification scheme meets certain defined criteria, someone holding the corresponding qualification will be recognised elsewhere
without a further test of competence.

The directives relating to doctors establish the requirements for
basic medical training and specialist qualification. The provisions
concerning basic medical training are straightforward and are being
used increasingly as seen by the growing numbers of junior hospital doctors in the UK who qualified in Germany or The

Netherlands. The situation regarding specialist qualification is more complicated as there are only some situations in which a specialist qualification is required, such as to be recognised for payment by a sickness fund in some countries (Brearley, 1995). None the less, the directives have been of considerable importance in the UK as they were one of the main factors behind the Calman reforms of medical education (Hunter & McLaren, 1993), which seek to ensure that British postgraduate medical training is compatible with that in the rest of Europe. It is arguable that this will come to be seen as one of the most important changes to the structure of the National Health Service since the 1960s as the smaller number of trainees available and the stricter criteria for training posts challenges the ability to provide a full range of services in some district general hospitals. Thus, while domestic health care is excluded from the competence of the European Union, it may be that a policy developed to ensure European harmonisation has major consequences for the NHS. Of course, this would not be the first example of this as the British government's policy of contracting out ancillary services was cast into disarray following the realisation that it was contrary to the TUPE (Transfer of Undertakings (Protection of Employment) directive) (Kline, 1993).

The situation concerning public health medicine is analogous to that in other specialities. The general principle is that free movement exists between any countries recognising that speciality. In the case of the major specialities, such as surgery, this typically includes all countries. Public health medicine is, however, only recognised in the United Kingdom, Ireland, France and Finland (McKee et al., 1992). In practice, free movement of health care professionals has been limited except where it is a continuation of historical patterns, such as between the UK and Ireland (Hurwitz, 1990). This is now changing, but formidable barriers remain.

IMPLICATIONS FOR RATIONING

There has been some concern that the freedom of movement of persons enshrined in the Treaties may limit the ability of national health bodies to set and enforce priorities. This would be the case if individuals had a right to obtain treatment anywhere in the Union. In fact, this right is somewhat limited. The main provisions, under the E111 system, provide only for those abroad for short stays to receive treatment that is immediately necessary and where the illness arose in the country of treatment. There are some minor exceptions, such as that to enable those on dialysis to travel freely. The right to travel abroad to receive treatment for a pre-existing condition (under the E112 system) is much more circumscribed as the responsible authority in the country of origin must give prior approval. There is one caveat. If a treatment is specified as an entitlement in national legislation, but cannot be provided within a reasonable time, then the authority must issue the approval. In the past, the vagueness of this provision and, specifically, the absence of a definition of 'reasonable time' has meant that this had little relevance. The British government may, however, inadvertently have changed the situation by introducing the Patient's Charter, which could be considered to have established 'reasonable times' to wait for treatment. This issue has recently received attention from patients' and consumers' groups and refusals to provide treatment abroad, where it is frequently much more easily available than in the UK, may now be open to legal challenge.

A related issue is the scope for health care providers to enter a system and offer, or induce demand for, services not currently provided. With the increasing pluralism in the NHS, in which health authorities and fundholders purchase from trusts, charities, and private providers, could purchasers be held in contempt of European competition law if they refuse to purchase services from a provider with its head office in another country? What would happen if a transnational chain attempted to penetrate the NHS internal market building hospitals which, after a period of predatory pricing, left them with a monopoly of hospital supply in some areas? The implications of the private finance initiative certainly create such a possibility so is the government lifting the lid of Pandora's box, only to have it flung open unexpectedly by European competition law? The situation is rather complicated although it has recently been reviewed in detail by Cohen (1994). On the basis of a ruling concerning education services, it seems likely that health services provided within a national system would not be considered 'services' in the meaning of the Treaties and thus would be exempt from competition law. This is, however, an area that requires continuing attention as it would be relatively easy to create the conditions in which health services do fall under the competence of competition law. In passing, it is useful to recall that European competition law already affects health care providers in that it requires that contracts above a certain threshold are advertised throughout the Union.

ELECTRONIC COMMUNICATION ACROSS FRONTIERS

The Data Protection Directive (European Commission, 1995), due to be implemented in the Member States by July 1997, establishes a single regulatory framework for the free movement of personal data throughout the EU. The proposed Directive for a Transparency Mechanism for Information Society Services (European Commission 1996) put forward by the Commission in July 1996, if finally adopted, would extend the scope of Directive 83/189 (which covers national rules affecting the free movement of goods) to include new Information Society services. The document defines 'Information Society Services' as all existing or new types of services that will be provided at a distance, by electronic means and on the individualised request of a service receiver including on-line health care services. However, the Directive would not require any harmonisation of the national rules, and would only seek to ensure that the single market is not fragmented and that no new regulatory barriers appear.

The Commission will ensure that national initiatives are compatible with freedom of establishment or free movement of services. As there is little movement of health services between member states so far, the relevance of the proposed Directive for health care is not immediately obvious. However, this is a rapidly changing area and, specifically, it may come to have important implications in the case of cross-border telemedicine care and private health insurance.

There is increasing interest and investment in the development of electronic systems that will support transnational health care provision. One example is the G7 Global Healthcare Application Project, which is also supported by the European Commission. This project involves a feasibility study evaluating the advantages of a global, interoperable health card. Several European pilot projects on health cards have been qualified successes, and G7 pilots are now planned that will evaluate a global emergency card and a global professional card.

Although the development of telemedicine in Europe is still in its infancy, it is expanding very rapidly and has important implications for the provision of cross-border health care. These include the development of computer-based patient records which will facilitate potential telemedicine applications at very low cost. Innovations currently being developed include radiology networks and applications in dermatology and pathology. More futuristic applications include robotic surgery.

The form that these developments will take will depend on several factors, including the further liberalisation of telecommunication services in Europe and the establishment of appropriate reimbursement methods. However, the establishment of the EC Information Society Programme and the new legislation on data transmission and data banks that is associated with it offers a framework for developing the innovations that will be required. Those involved in this programme are looking to developments in the USA. For example, the US Health Care Financing Administration has recently introduced a three-year trial of Medicare reimburse ment for teleconsultations involving 'hub' hospitals and distance 'spokes'. The project is running in four states (Georgia, Iowa, North Carolina and West Virginia) and it is expected that it will lead to federal enabling legislation within five years (Anon, 1997).

DEVELOPMENTS IN PRIVATE HEALTH INSURANCE

Changes in rules on data protection also have implications for cross-border provision of private health insurance, but here the most important factor is the third Insurance Directives which introduced important changes in the insurance market in the European Union.

In the past, there have been two main models for the supervision of insurance operations in the member states. The first is known as material regulation and the second is based on financial regulation. The former exists in Germany where regulation is based on the idea that, if insurers are sufficiently controlled in the type of business that they undertake and the level of premiums they charge, there can be no question of insolvency. The supervisory body considers the policies before they are offered on sale. In addition, in Germany, only insurers who specialise in health care can operate in the field of private health insurance to protect policyholders from insolvency arising from other business. The second model was implemented in the UK. According to this model, the regulator assesses solvency on the basis of annual accounts, leaving the detailed managemnt of policies to the insurer. The transposition into national law of the third Insurance Directives has a substantial effect on the so-called common insurance area. The major consequence for the UK will be that insurers incorporated in any member state can conduct business throughout the European Union, subject only to regulation in their home state. This raises the question of the regulatory ability of the member states to monitor the activities of insurance firms operating in their jurisdictions (Mossialos & Le Grand, 1997).

DEVELOPMENTS IN MAIL-ORDER DISPENSING

A related area that may be affected by European integration is mail-order dispensing of drugs. Cross-border dispensing is not expected to grow significantly in the near future because of the lack of harmonisation of the relevant laws and the major differences in national reimbursement systems. There are, however, some emerging issues that could change this, not least the interest in direct sales by the pharmaceutical industry. For example, in the USA in 1992, mail-order sales accounted for 6.8% of the total pharmaceutical market. The present situation is that there have been two judgements by the European Court of Justice, one involving over-the-counter drugs and the other prescription only drugs. Both reaffirmed the rights of individuals to import by post reasonable quantities of a medicine for their own use. The European Commission also argues that the directives on movement of doctors preclude the refusal to honour a prescription on the grounds that a prescribing doctor is a foreign national or lives in another member state (Anon, 1993). This is an area that is still somewhat contentious and the British General Medical Council argues that prescriptions are only valid in the UK if they are written by doctors registered with it.

BSE AND THE POWER TO LIMIT TRADE

As noted above, the world-wide ban on the export of British beef following the announcement that the British Spongiform Encephalopathy Advisory Committee had taken the view that consumption of infected beef was the most likely cause of ten cases of new variant Creutzfeld–Jakob Disease has had enormous political and financial implications. Consequently, it is appropriate to examine briefly the basis for this action. A more detailed discussion of the specific legal issues raised in the BSE case appears elsewhere (McKee & Steyger, 1997).

In brief, free movement of goods means that countries are unable to restrict imports except in narrowly defined circumstances, one of which is concern about public health. The circumstances in which this argument can be used has been clarified following a landmark case in which Germany was found to have acted unlawfully in blocking the import of a liqueur, Cassis de Dijon. The court ruled that, in principle, a product lawfully marketed and produced in one member state must be allowed into another member state unless it can be shown that a ban is part of a 'seriously considered public health policy', is proportional to the objective being pursued, the objective could not be achieved in another way, and be shown to be both necessary to protect health and goes no further than is necessary. The court has, however, recognised that there are often differences of opinion on the nature and magnitude of public health risks and seems willing to veer on the side of those who can show that there is genuine doubt about safety. Thus it seems likely that the recent ban on the import of genetically engineered maize by the Austrian government, which is contrary to a decision made by the Commission, would be considered legal.

These examples show that domestic policies, even in areas which do not, at first sight, appear to have any European dimension, may turn out to fall within the competence of European law

SPECIFIC POLICIES ON PUBLIC HEALTH

Formally, the scope for action by the European Union in the area of public health is limited. First, the treaties give it specific competence in only a few areas related to public health. Secondly, many areas of health and health care are covered by the concept of subsidiarity, in which issues should be dealt with at the lowest appropriate level, a concept interpreted in the UK as meaning at national level but in most other countries extending to regional and local level. To elaborate this concept, the 1992 Edinburgh summit introduced a three stage test for future legislation. First, has the Community competence to act? Secondly, if it does have competence, is it impossible to achieve the desired objectives at national level? And thirdly, if measures are not attainable at national level, what is the minimum Community intervention necessary? However, this leaves ample scope for differing national perspectives (Watson, 1994a; Schleicher, 1994) with the former British government under John Major adopting a very narrow interpretation.

As noted earlier, for the first time, the Maastricht Treaty gave the European Union specific competence in the field of public health. Article 129 enables the European Union to take action to co-ordinate national policies on the prevention of major diseases, including drug dependence, as well as health information and education.

This Article is the responsibility of Directorate General (DG) V, (Employment, Industrial Relations and Social Affairs). The scope for action is limited and the Union may only provide incentives for action or, through a qualified majority vote in the Council, adopt a recommendation proposed by the Commission.

It is important to note that the way Article 129 is worded emphasises prevention of major diseases rather than the broader promotion of health. Its implementation reflects this, although there is a recognition in the Commission of the importance of policies that address the broader determinants of health (Watson, 1994b). As the issuance of directives or regulations is precluded, the scope for changing national policies is limited but as the ability to take 'incentive measures', when supported by funds, taken with the requirement on the Commission to 'any useful initiative' to ensure that Member States should co-ordinate their policies makes it likely that national policies will increasingly be influenced by decisions made at a European level as new developments supported under such programmes will comply with common objectives.

In 1993, the European Commission published a resolution setting out a framework for future action in the field of public health that would provide a basis for implementing the provisions of the treaty in respect of public health (European Commission, 1993). It accepted that 'public health policy as such, except in cases where the Treaties provide otherwise, is the responsibility of the Member States', but argued for the need for a mechanism by which the member states and the Commission could consult and collaborate. It also highlighted the need to develop a long-term approach to public health issues and established certain criteria for Community action. These are that there is a significant health problem and appropriate preventive actions are possible; the aim of the activity cannot be sufficiently achieved by the Member States acting alone; the activity supplements or promotes other Community policies such as the operation of the single market; and that the activity is consistent with those of other international organisations, such as the World Health Organisation. It continued by noting the need for better data to inform priority setting and identified criteria to be used in setting priorities, such as mortality, morbidity, years of life impaired and cost. Specific actions proposed in the framework documents were confined to establishing a high-level committee of representatives of Member States, exchange of information through networks of institutions specialising in particular areas and exchange of personnel, establishment of mechanisms to ensure that health policy is taken into account in other European Union policies, and mechanisms for improved co-operation with international organisations.

While this framework sets out the overall direction of future activity, there is also a series of other programmes, some of which predate the Maastricht Treaty. These include the Europe against

Cancer and Europe against AIDS programmes as well as programmes on drugs and other specific challenges to health. These are
described in the following paragraphs. The current levels of funding are given in Table 4.1.

Table 4.1   Funding for EU health related programmes

Programme	Funding (million ecu)
Europe against AIDS (1996–1999)	49.6
Europe against Cancer (1996–2000)	64
Health promotion, information and training (1996–1999)	35
Prevention of drug dependence (1996–2000)	28.5
Health and safety at work (1996–2000)	66
Safety action in Europe (1996–2000)	41.5
European home and leisure accident surveillance (1994–1997)	11
European Agency for Health and Safety at Work	n/a

In 1988, the European Community adopted the Europe against
Cancer programme, (European Commission, 1988) with an initial
annual budget of 10 million ecus. It includes campaigns against
tobacco, improvements in nutrition, protection against carcinogenic
agents, promotion of screening policies, the provision of information
to the public and professionals, and research. The third phase of the
Europe against Cancer programme (1996–2000) focuses on four areas:

• data collection and research;
• information and health education;
• early detection and screening; and
• training and quality control.

One of the programme's aims is to identify cancer research requirements at European level and to support the creation of an inventory of cancer research in progress.

In 1991, a similar programme, 'Europe against AIDS', was adopted, encompassing the provision of information and training,
exchange of information on services, research, and measures to promote the safety of blood. The 1996–1999 phase of the Europe
against AIDS programme focuses on the following activities:

• surveillance and monitoring of communicable diseases;
• combating transmission;

- information, education and training and support for persons with HIV/AIDS; and
- combating discrimination.

The European Home and Leisure Accident and Surveillance System aims to support and complement actions being implemented by the member states by identifying the products involved in accidents and the combination of circumstances which might lead to these accidents. The European Commission is responsible for processing and disseminating at European level the data collected by the member states.

The Commission has also introduced the Community action programme on the prevention of drug dependence within the framework for action in the field of public health, 1996–2000. The aim is to co-ordinate and promote intra-Community co-operation and measures to stimulate member states' own efforts to prevent drug addiction. Emphasis will be placed on improving knowledge of the phenomenon of drug dependence and its consequences, and of the methods of preventing drug addiction. In addition, activities will focus on prevention of drug dependence and improving awareness of the associated risks, in particular, for young people and especially vulnerable groups.

Research programmes are already directed at nutrition, cardiovascular diseases, mental illness and the problems associated with ageing. The Commission is now preparing draft communications and proposals for European Parliament-Council decisions concerning five year action programmes on rare diseases, pollution-related diseases and the prevention of injuries. It has also prepared drafts with a view to adoption in 1997 of proposals concerning safety and self-sufficiency of blood. The development of methodologies and capacity for the evaluation of health and health-related programmes is foreseen by the health monitoring programme and preparatory work has already been carried out (Holland & Mossialos, 1997).

The EU has also been active in developing global collaboration in the field of public health. In May 1996, the United States government and the European Commission established a joint US–EU Task Force to develop a global early warning system for communicable diseases under the Transatlantic Agenda. The Task Force is to develop a unified pragmatic and flexible surveillance and response network for communicable diseases, with global geographic coverage.

The European Commission has also established a Task Force for Vaccines within the Directorate General for Research, The Task Force published its first report in December 1995 and proposed amongst others, to:

- establish a European partnership between governments, industry and academia on common projects in vaccines R&D;
- establish general criteria for the identification of priorities;
- concentrate efforts in vaccine research and co-ordination of policies within the EC by creating a co-ordinated flow of information concerning the relevant activities of different specific programmes;
- create networks of scientific resources for optimising strategies in vaccine research;
- concentrate European R&D of new and improved vaccines on the preventive and therapeutic means for the control of the major viral diseases and other infectious and chronic diseases; and
- develop vaccine delivery systems and their specificity for the induction of different arms of the immune system.

As the above examples show, the European Union has moved in a relatively short period from a situation in which it had little involvement in public health to one in which it has become a major player in international health. Most of these programmes are still at a very early stage, but it is likely that they will have an increasingly important influence on the development of national health policies.

NEW EUROPEAN AGENCIES

In addition to the above policies, the European Union has recently established a series of specialised agencies that have relevance for public health and health care.

In 1993, the European Union established the European Medicines Evaluation Agency, in London. Member states have lost their regulatory powers in the field of biotechnology. The agency also has competence in authorising innovative pharmaceutical products. It is important to note that the driving force behind the creation of this agency was the industry, who are anxious to develop the single European market. This is in contrast to the American Food and Drugs Administration, whose establishment was the result of consumer pressure in the wake of the Thalidomide affair. The agency was established by the Commissioner with responsibility for Industrial Policy and there was no involvement by the Directorate responsible for Social Affairs, including public health. The relationship between the agency and the national regulatory agencies, although apparently clear, still has some unresolved issues, not least the absence of an agreed definition of innovation, unlike the situation in the USA.

The consequences of drug addiction have been a major preoccupation of member states and there is widespread agreement on the need for international action. To reflect these views, the Commission developed an action programme covering the period up to the year 2000. In addition, the European Drugs and Drugs Addiction Monitoring Centre was established in Lisbon in 1993 (Council of Ministers, 1993). The priorities of the Centre include collection of reliable and comparable data and exchange of information. Its initial priority is the study of demand for drugs and its reduction. It co-ordinates a European information network known as REITOX (réseau européan d'information sur la toxicomanie).

The European Environment Agency, established in Copenhagen, is responsible for producing objective, reliable and comparable information necessary for drawing up and implementing future EU environmental policies and for ensuring public awareness about the environment. The agency is in a key position to undertake research on the environmental determinants of health and to link environmental and health data. Its work programme for 1994–1999 includes the study of threats to human health by means of a continuously updated databank.

In 1994 the Commision established the European Agency for Health and Safety at Work. It is responsible for providing technical, scientific and economic information for use in the field of health and safety at work. Its activities include promoting and supporting co-operation through exchange of information and experience among the member states, and establishing networks, with particular attention to the problems faced by small and medium enterprises.

The agencies are still in their infancy, but they are likely to play an increasing role in European health policy formation. The European Medicines Evaluation Agency is the only one with regulatory powers and the others are limited to co-ordination, collection of data, and exchange of information. These are, however, extremely important roles.

RESEARCH POLICY

There was no provision for research in the Treaty of Rome which established the European Economic Community. The Member States could interpret Article 235 of the Treaty to develop policies in the field of research but this did not happen until 1974. The 1987 Single European Act introduced Title VI on Research and Technological Development, subsequently amended by the Maastricht Treaty. This states that 'the Community shall have the objective of strengthening the scientific and technological basis of Community industry and encouraging it to become more competitive at international level, while promoting all the research activities deemed necessary by virtue of other Chapters of this Treaty'. It is evident that economic preoccupations are the underlying premises of the Treaty, but the final words provide the opportunity to the Community to develop research activities in other areas not directly related with industrial competitiveness.

The Maastricht Treaty expanded the scope of research by introducing the legal basis for the Framework Research Programmes. These programmes should reflect the stated scientific and technological priorities of the Treaty, indicate the general focus of such activities and define the amount of financial support available and the detailed rules for financial participation by the Community.

Research Framework Programmes are adopted by the co-decision procedure described above. Unanimity is required in the Council and the European Parliament has power to reject the whole Programme. However, the European Parliament cannot reject only part of the Programme or amend parts of it. A detailed negotiation procedure follows after the submission of the Commission's proposals.

The first Medical and Health Research Programme (MHR) was adopted by the Council of Ministers in 1978. This was followed by MHR 2, 3 and 4 programmes, which were succeeded by the first and the second Biomedical and Health Research Programmes (BIO-MED 1 and BIOMED 2). Table 4.2 illustrates the evolution of the EC health related programmes between 1978 and 1998 (Baert, 1995). It is evident that the growth of research funding between 1978 and 1994 was considerable and has resulted in a significant increase of projects sponsored and research teams involved. However, an evaluation of the effectiveness of these programmes has not been undertaken and it is not clear that their results have had any significant impact on policy formation at either EU or national level.

Table 4.2   Evolution of European Union biomedical and health research

Programme	Budget (million ecu)	Scope	Participation
MHR 1 (1978–81)	1.09	3 concerted actions	100 teams
MHR 2 (1980–83)	2.32	7 concerted actions	230 teams
MHR 3 (1982–86)	13.3	34 concerted actions	1200 teams
MHR 4 (1987–91)	65	135 concerted actions	4540 teams
BIOMED 1 (1990–94)	133	362 concerted actions and 41 shared cost projects	7300 teams
BIOMED 2 (1994–98)	358	n/a	n/a

The current programme, BIOMED 2, focuses on seven target areas:

● pharmaceutical research;
● research on biomedical technology and engineering;
● brain research;
● diseases with major socio-economic impact;
● human genome research;
● public health research;
● research on biomedical ethics.

The first call for proposals, which closed on 31st March 1995, attracted 1709 proposals from some 6000 organisations.

European Union research on health and related areas is now playing a significant part in overall health research funding.

LEARNING FROM EXPERIENCE

Closer European integration is also affecting public health policies through the accelerated diffusion of knowledge of the differences in health between countries and regions of Europe and the varying policy responses to health challenges. Life expectancy at birth in the countries of Western Europe varies by almost five years (WHO, 1996). If the countries of Central and Eastern Europe are included, the differences are even greater. These figures conceal even greater variation in the pattern of disease, with some countries, such as the United Kingdom and Ireland, experiencing very high levels of ischaemic heart diseases, while Portugal has an exceptionally high death rate from cerebrovascular disease, and Danish women are especially likely to die from lung cancer. Furthermore, these patterns are changing over time and in different directions, with some countries achieving reductions in deaths from conditions such as ischaemic heart disease and lung cancer, while in others they continue to increase. On even closer inspection, the differences remain with, for example, the United Kingdom having a particularly good record on overall deaths from road traffic accidents, but one of the worst in Europe if only children under five are considered.

These differences highlight the need for public health professionals to place the health of their local population in a wider European perspective as, if they do not do so, they will fail to recognise the possibilities for change. Fortunately, these observations have stimulated a body of research, much of which is funded by the European Commission, to explore the reasons for these differences and the impact of the various national policies adopted in response to particular health challenges. A few examples will illustrate some of the insights that have been gained. As this is written largely for a British audience, the examples concentrate on situations in which this country has room for improvement rather than those areas such as communicable disease control (Desenclos *et al.*, 1993) and sleeping position and sudden infant death (McKee *et al.*, 1996c) in which the UK is ahead of many other European countries.

The observation that southern European countries had much longer life expectancies than would be predicted given their economic development led to a recognition that this could largely be attributed to their very low rates of ischaemic heart disease. The research that arose from this observation has now led to a recognition of the importance of a 'Mediterranean diet' (de Lorgeril *et al.*, 1994). This, in turn, has stimulated a large volume of research on the relationship between diet, and in particular fresh fruit and vegetables and alcohol. Although all the details of this complex issue have not yet been disentangled, the findings so far have already influenced national nutritional policies throughout Europe, and the resulting dietary changes seem likely to have contributed to the fall in deaths from ischaemic heart disease seen in Northern Europe in recent years.

Death rates increase in most countries in winter, but the rise in the UK is the highest in Europe. Indeed, the increase is almost nonexistent in some Nordic countries with much colder winters than the UK (McKee, 1989). This has focused attention on the relatively poor standard of the housing stock in the UK and has led to a major collaborative project on the effect of indoor temperature on mortality (Eurowinter Group, 1997).

The teenage pregnancy rate in the UK is now the highest in the

European Union, at 31.8 live births per 1000 females aged 15–19 in 1992. The next highest level, in Austria, is only 23.1 and that in The Netherlands, which has the lowest rate, is only 5.8 (Council of Europe, 1994). This strongly suggests that it may be possible to learn from the way in which sex education and access to contraceptive services are provided in The Netherlands. The open approach adopted by the Dutch contrasts markedly with that in the UK, in which some years ago sex education materials were withdrawn on the orders of a minister as they were deemed to be too explicit.

Although, overall, there are fewer deaths from road traffic accidents in the UK than in many neighbouring countries, as noted above, this is not true of deaths among young children, where the rate is among the highest. Those countries that have much better records have often implemented large-scale traffic calming measures in residential areas and taken steps to ensure that children and vehicles are physically separated, while permitting both to use open spaces (Ruxton, 1996). One of the consequences of the policies adopted in the UK has been to force children indoors during play and into cars as they travel around (Hillman, 1990). For example, one survey found that 60% of journeys made by Dutch children between 12 and 15 were by bicycle, whereas the corresponding figure for the UK was only 6% (European Parliament, 1991). The health consequences of these differences are potentially far reaching, compounded by the situation whereby, as a result of selling playing fields and curriculum changes, the number of hours spent on physical activity in British schools is also the lowest in Europe.

The last example is arguably an indicator of the more general problem of the low status of children in the UK compared with other European countries, characterised by the Victorian dictum that 'children should be seen but not heard'. This has been exacerbated by the introduction of market based policies in the 1980s and 1990s in the UK, USA, Australia and New Zealand but not in most continental countries. The consequences have been catalogued in a UNICEF report which shows how, for example, using an index of social health of children, the situation in the Anglo-Saxon countries has been deteriorating while it improved on the continent (Hewlett, 1993).

In addition to the insights available on specific health challenges, a European perspective may also contribute to a better understanding of the global determinants of health at national level. The limited ability of individual risk factors to explain differences in health, as shown by research like the Whitehall study, is focusing interest on population level variables (Davey Smith *et al.*, 1994). The large variation in life expectancy at birth within the European Union, almost 5 years for men and 2.5 years for women in 1990, offers many opportunities for research (Abel-Smith *et al.*, 1995). A recent example that illustrates this issue arises from a study that sought to explain why life expectancy has stagnated in Denmark over the last two decades. A comparison with the situation in Sweden showed that this reflected either a failure to achieve the same improvements or an actual deterioration in death rates from almost all causes, suggesting a fundamental underlying problem in Danish society not explained by known risk factors (Chenet *et al.*, 1996a). Looking further afield, research on health in central and eastern Europe is shedding light on the widespread health consequences of high levels of alcohol consumption, which may have relevance in the countries of Western Europe (Chenet *et al.*, 1996b).

Of course, the existence of different health policies does not imply necessarily that those in place elsewhere can simply be imported. Those seeking to transfer ideas must recognise national differences in historical, cultural, geographical and economic context.

CONCLUSIONS

European integration is having an increasing impact on many aspects of public health practice and research. The consequences of developments in European law, not only where it is obviously related to health but also in areas such as health and safety, trade, and competition policy are of increasing importance to those involved in developing and implementing public health policy at national level. Consequently, it is of the greatest importance that these developments, and the ways in which they arise, are understood. Increasingly, it will be essential that the public health perspective is brought to bear on legislation as it is being developed within the bodies of the European Union. At present, this process is still something of a mystery to many people, a situation encouraged by the minimal media coverage of European affairs by the British media, the unwritten policy of the former government to marginalise the British members of the European Parliament, and the conspicuous failure of the Houses of Commons and Lords to scrutinise adequately European legislation at a time when it could be changed. There have now been several examples of how the UK can find its scope for action unexpectedly constrained due to failure to consid-

er the consequences of European law. The example of the data protection directive, where the public health community suceeded in
ensuring that epidemiological research was not prevented, is a rare,
if extremely successful, example of how effective pressure can be
brought to bear (Smith, 1996).

Similarly, it is increasingly important for researchers and practitioners to look to the experiences of others. A narrow national focus,
which seeks only to compare local achievements in public health
with the best in the UK, may provide some reassurance but, as
noted above, can often lead to acceptance of mediocrity and a failure to recognise what can be achieved. In every European country
there is scope to learn from the experience of someone else, who will
be doing things differently. In addition, as there is wider recognition of the magnitude of the differences in health between countries, researchers will increasingly focus their efforts on explaining
why these exist.

REFERENCES

Abel-Smith B, Figueras J, Holland W, McKee M, Mossialis E 1995 Choices in
    Health Policy: An agenda for the European Union. Dartmouth Press/ Office for
    Official Publications of the European Communities, Aldershot/ Luxembourg
Anon 1993 Prescriptions valid throughout EC says EC Commissioner.
    Pharmaceutical Journal May 8: 628
Anon 1997 Telemedicine: Big sister is watching you. The Economist 11th January:
    51
Baert AE 1995 History of medical research at EC level. In European Union
    Biomedical and Health Research: The Biomed 1 Programme. AE Baert, SS Baig,
    C Bardoux et al. ed. IOS Press, Amsterdam
Brearley S 1995 Harmonisation of specialist training in Europe: is it a mirage?
    British Medical Journal 311: 297–9
Chapman S 1991 Europe's chance to ban tobacco advertising. British Journal of
    Addiction 86: 1383–5
Chenet L, Osler M, McKee M, Krasnik A 1996a Changing life expectancy in the
    1980s: why was Denmark different from Sweden? Journal of Epidemiology and
    Community Health 50: 404–7
Chenet L, McKee M, Fulop N et al 1996b Changing life expectancy in central
    Europe: is there a single reason? Journal of Public Health Medicine 18: 329–36
Cohen, P 1994 The separation of purchaser from provider in health care systems
    and European Community law: The case of the British National Health Service.
    LSE Health Discussion paper No 1. LSE Health, London
Council of Europe 1994 Recent Demographic Developments in Europe. Council of
    Europe, Strasbourg
Council of Ministers 1993 Council Regulation (EEC) No 302/93 establishing a
    European Monitoring Centre on Drugs and Drugs Addiction, Official Journal of
    the European Communities, L 36
Davey Smith G, Blane D, Bartley M 1994 Explanations for socio-economic differ-
    entials in mortality: evidence from Britain and elsewhere. European Journal of
    Public Health 4: 131–4

de Lorgeril M, Renaud S, Mamelle N et al 1994 Mediterranean alpha-linoleic acid rich diet in secondary prevention of coronary heart disease. Lancet 343: 1454–9
Desenclos J-C, Bijkerk H, Huisman J 1993 Variations in national infectious disease surveillance in Europe. Lancet 341: 1003–6
European Commission 1988 Decision 88–351 of the Council adopting a 1988 to 1989 plan of action for an information and public awareness campaign in the context of the 'Europe against cancer' programme. Official Journal of the European Communities C184/05
European Commission 1993 Council Resolution on future action in the field of public health. Official Journal of the European Communities C 174/1
European Commission 1995 Directive 95/46/EC on the protection of the individual with regard to the processing of personal data and the free movement of such data. Official Journal of the European Communities L281
European Commission 1996 Communication from the Commission to the European Parliament, the Council and the Economic and Social Committee concerning regulatory transparency in the internal market for information society services. COM (96) 392 final. European Commission, Brussels
European Parliament 1991 Committee on Youth, Culture, Education, the Media and Sport. Report on the problems of children in the European Community A3–0000/91. European Parliament, Strasbourg
Eurowinter Group 1997 Cold exposure and winter mortality from ischaemic heart disease, cerebrovascular disease, respiratory disease, and all causes in warm and cold regions of Europe. Lancet 349: 1341–6
Hewlett SA 1993 Child Neglect in Rich Nations. UNICEF, New York
Hillman M 1990 One false move ... a study of children's independent mobility. Policy Studies Institute, London
Holland W Mossialos E 1997 Public Health Decisions: Methods of Priority Setting in the EU Member States, Office for Official Publications of the European Communities, 1997, Luxembourg
Hunter S, McLaren P 1993 Specialist medical training and the Calman report. British Medical Journal 306: 1281–2.
Hurwitz L 1990 The Free Circulation of Physicians Within the European Community. Avebury, Aldershot
Jenkins S 1995 Accountable to None: The Tory nationalisation of Britain. Hamish Hamilton, London
Kline R 1993 TUPE: Safe transfer. Health Visitor 66: 377
Marr A 1995 Ruling Britannia: The failure and future of British democracy. Michael Joseph, London
McKee CM 1989 Deaths in winter: can Britain learn from Europe? European Journal of Epidemiology 5: 178–82
McKee M, Clarke A, Kornitzer M, et al 1992 Public health medicine training in the European Community: is there scope for harmonization? European Journal of Public Health 2: 45–53
McKee M, Lang T, Roberts J 1996a Deregulating health: policy lessons of the BSE affair. Journal of the Royal Society of Medicine 89: 424–6
McKee M, Mossialos E, Belcher P 1996b The impact of European Union law on national health policy. Journal of European Social Policy 6: 263–86.
McKee M, Fulop N, Bouvier P et al 1996c Preventing sudden infant deaths — the slow diffusion of an idea. Health Policy 37: 117–35
McKee M, Steyger E. When can the European Union restrict trade on grounds of public health? Journal of Public Health Medicine 1997 (forthcoming)
Mossialos E, Le Grand J 1997. Cost containment in health care in the fifteen EU member states. Office for Official Publications of the European Communities, Luxembourg
Ruxton S 1996 Children in Europe. NCH Action for Children, London
Schleicher, U. 1994 European health policy before and after Maastricht. In Cost

Containment, Pricing and Financing of Pharmaceuticals in the European Community: The policy makers' view. ed. E. Mossialos, C. Ranos C, B. Abel-Smith. Pharmetrica, Athens

Smith M F 1996 Data protection, health care, and the new European directive British Medical Journal 312: 197–8

Watson R. 1994a What the new European parliament might do about health. British Medical Journal 308: 1392

Watson R. 1994b European Union puts health at centre of new policy. British Medical Journal 308: 1530

Weatherill S, Beamont P 1996 EC Law. Penguin, Harmondsworth, pp 337–82

WHO 1996 Health for All database. Copenhagen, WHO

5. The Role of Theory in Public Health

Ian Jones and Drew Walker

INTRODUCTION

In this chapter we revisit four papers published in the early 1980s on the place of theory in public health and the implications for its practice of various theoretical approaches (Cameron & Jones, 1982, 1983, 1985; Jones & Cameron, 1984), respond here to some of the issues raised, comment on public health theoretical analysis since then and reassemble the arguments into an updated position.

THEORY IN PUBLIC HEALTH

The first of these papers (Cameron & Jones, 1982) remarked on the importance of doctors, particularly those in public health, having a theory of society. In contrast to other sciences, where philosophy and theory are an integral part, medical practitioners rarely give any indication of the theoretical basis of their practice and generally ignore social factors in health. However, there are areas of medical practice in which theory does arise where the underlying hypotheses are not dependent on a sociological analysis. First, they exist in pre-clinical subjects such as anatomy, physiology and pharmacology. Secondly, in epidemiology there is much commentary on arcane technical aspects of the subject. Thirdly, there is a plethora of hypotheses which characterise public health and which are inaccurately referred to as theories. Finally, in the absence of specific social theories, there are ideologies, or hidden theories, which exist as unspoken beliefs.

Ideology functions at the subconscious rather than at the conscious level. It is a system of representations, images, myths, ideas or concepts endowed with a historical existence and role within any given society. It is able to present a false picture of reality in an internally consistent, logical and acceptable form. It creates a system of beliefs which make the most absurd propositions appear intellectually acceptable at a certain level. It is remarkably resistant to change, even in the face of scientific knowledge, and has its sources in the law, religion, politics, the arts, literature and other areas of our culture. It imbues every aspect of our lives and is expressed through political and other leaders, role models, friends, television, radio and other media, and most obviously through political propaganda and advertising.

In default of a social theory public health doctors are often eclectic and consequently inconsistent. The authors' position as Marxists, or materialists, led them to believe that, since health is socially determined by the material world, the product of changing circumstances and individual action, medicine in general and public health in particular should be practised by means of changing society.

Cameron and Jones then presented a critique of four ideologies prevalent amongst practitioners of public health: idealism, social Darwinism, objectivism and empiricism.

Idealism is a set of beliefs involving a tendency to regard humans as free-floating, cocooned from society's influence and unaffected by the material world. In this asocial theory, ill-health results from individuals spontaneously adopting what medical experts see as perverse patterns of behaviour which bring about their own destruction. At a time when the existence of society is being questioned, examples are to be found in official government documents and are commonplace in the annual reports of Chief Medical Officers and some Directors of Public Health. Their views can be paraphrased as, 'If only people were to stop smoking and drinking, have sex with only one person, start eating sensibly, and take responsibility for their own health, then they would be healthy.' Quasi-religious homilies to mend one's ways offer a very limited kind of health education and cannot tackle problems which have their real origins not in the actions of the individuals but in the nature of our society. The authors' apparent over-riding need is to avoid upsetting any of the organisations, be they the government ministers or departments, health or local authorities, or independent bodies, principally responsible for creating the circumstances that lead to ill-health in the first place. A rejection of the view that behaviours such as smoking can be freely chosen, and hence a critique of idealism, does appear in the public health literature from time to time (Cornell & Milner, 1996).

Social Darwinism is the inappropriate application of the biological principles of survival of the fittest to human behaviour and social systems. It is the pseudo-scientific justification of the politics of discrimination on grounds of race, sex, religion, disability, poverty and disadvantage according to the 'laws of nature'. It had its origins last century in Malthus, Spencer and Galton, and would probably be more accurately described as Galtonism. Although few medical people today would admit publicly to subscribing to it in its most overt and repugnant 'eugenic' form, the views of racist ideologues re-emerge from time to time and are then subjected to critique in the scientific press (Mackintosh, 1996). A concise yet trenchant critique of the theory has recently been published (Burry, 1996). The theory is based on false reasoning: first that natural selection works on genes rather than whole animals living in their communities; secondly, that it is possible to reduce all life to the action of genes or any other single principle (reductionism); and thirdly, that humans are passive victims of nature. In reality, deliberate social policies, including education, health, family planning, housing and control of communicable diseases by immunisation are now responsible for some of the most important attributes in society.

Objectivism is the tendency to adopt an extra-world view of society in which humans are treated akin to laboratory animals. A humorous version of this view is presented in *The Hitch-hiker's Guide to the Galaxy*. Stress is laid upon what is objective or external to the mind. Objectivism must be distinguished from being objective, the latter being an essential element of separating ourselves from the results of scientific work. Objectivism attempts to step so far back from scientific work as to suggest we are in no way involved. Science, far from being neutral, is a human activity which should not attempt to place the interests of the state, communities, corporations or populations above the interests of individual people. The function of public health is to determine the needs of people by reference to them and their representatives, consulting and entering into dialogue with them to reach agreement on their health care needs. The objectivist tendency either ignores this consultative stage, or pays lip service to it, arguing that the issues are too complex for 'non-experts' to participate in meaningfully. It is inappropriate in a democratic society for medical people or any other professional group on their own to attempt to determine priorities. Equally inappropriate are applications of economic evaluation which seek to balance the costs to an organisation with the benefits to an individual. Only where both costs and benefits are borne by the same individual or organisation can they be judged for that individual or organisation. These difficulties can be addressed only when those practising public health treat individuals as participants rather than objects. Recent publicity in the United Kingdom on the refusal of an English health authority to fund intensive chemotherapy and a second bone marrow transplant in a child with leukaemia fuelled this debate. Whether the health authority took the decision with the best of motives and in the best interests of the child, as it claimed, cannot be known for certain. Nevertheless, this case illustrates the difficulty faced by society in reconciling conflicting views of individuals and organisations although a purely objectivist approach to resolving this conflict remains inappropriate.

Empiricism is the theory which rejects the need for theory; it relates all knowledge to what our experience and senses tell us. It is the concentration on facts, or what passes for them, to the exclusion of theory. It is the sociology of the obvious — everything is what it seems. As such, it must be distinguished from empirical observations which are part and parcel of science. Empiricism is so widespread in epidemiology as to be commonplace; virtually nothing can be described without it being analysed in the UK by age, sex and social class, and in the USA by age, sex and race. This is done without any thought to its relevance to understanding the problem at hand. Most texts on epidemiology fail to convey the impression of real men and women functioning in society or to analyse the real social structures within which we live. The groupings, generally called 'variables', appear to be chosen more for their convenience than their value.

EMPIRICISM

The second and third papers in the series by Cameron and Jones dealt more fully with the last of these ideologies, empiricism.

In the second, the empiricist approach of modern epidemiological texts was examined using the example of John Snow and the Broad Street pump (Cameron & Jones, 1983). This paper discussed Snow's theories and actions and described how modern texts have inaccurately characterised the nature of his contribution to the understanding and control of the cholera outbreak in 1854. Whereas Snow is widely credited with the removal of the pump handle, the cessation of the outbreak and with the identification of the source, in fact he did none of these. The first was carried out by local parishioners, the outbreak was subsiding before the pump handle was removed and the third was identified by his friend and collaborator, the Reverend Henry Whitehead. Snow's genius lay in the application of all his skills and knowledge, medical, sociological, mathematical, political and economic to the problem. His theory was that cholera was caused by living, reproducing micro-organisms which affect people most commonly in conditions of poverty. The spread of cholera by contaminated water was not his theory: rather it was a deduction from it. Whereas modern epidemiologists have concentrated on his statistical skills Snow used these only to help build up the case for the theory he had already developed, one which took germ theory as far as was possible at the time before the advent of bacteriology.

It is important to ask why Snow's work on cholera was ignored at the time by all the medical and other authorities of the day and is regularly misinterpreted today. He received no credit for his work on cholera until resurrected by Wade Hampton Frost in the 1930s, some 80 years after his death, possibly because his technical methods and succinct writing fitted in well with 20th century, essentially empiricist, numerical approaches to epidemiology.

Snow believed that cholera was caused by a self-replicating organism which could be spread by contagion. Since quarantine was the only known method of containing contagious diseases at the time and this conflicted with the political and economic necessity of the industrial and capitalist revolution, medical men may have therefore been, consciously or subconsciously, more inclined to support the multifactorial miasmatic theory of von Pettenkoffer than the nascent germ theory of Snow. Certainly official documents of the time made it quite clear that: '...there is no one point on which medical men are so clearly agreed as on the connexion of exposure of persons to the miasma from sewers and of fever as a consequence' (Poor Law Commissioners, 1842). The extent to which political considerations lay behind the rejection of Snow by the then medical establishment is unknown, although there seems little doubt that it played a significant role with some of them.

The third paper addressed the issue of social class, describing its concept and derivation as an embarrassment to epidemiology (Jones & Cameron, 1984). In its modern form it owes its origin to Thomas Henry Craig Stevenson, Superintendent of Statistics in the General Register Office, London, from 1909 until 1931. He had already reached the conclusion by 1913 that '...in so far as infantile mortality depends upon social position it may be expected to be lowest in Class 1 and to increase regularly down to Class 5...' (Registrar General, 1913). When he subsequently discovered 'discrepancies' in the Supplement to the 75th Annual Report (Registrar General, 1923), he solved the problem neatly by making '...a very moderate assumption to suppose that 10% of the mortality credited to Class V properly belongs to Class IV', and promptly knocked 10% off the figures at every age group for the former and added them to the latter (Stevenson, 1923). Although in their defence of social class analysis Leete and Fox (1977) have claimed that the 1911 classification was not designed by reference to infant mortality rates of occupational groups, Stevenson made sure that the revisions for which he was responsible certainly were by moving occupational groups from one class to another to meet his mortality expectations. Szreter (1984) points out that Stevenson may also have modified or manipulated the classification using fertility data. Stevenson made no attempt to hide his manipulations and his actions were in no way comparable to the fraud perpetrated by Gregor Mendel and others. Nevertheless, the overall effect was the same; the result became part of the general body of knowledge to the exclusion of the illegitimate means of attaining it. In Mendel's case history has confirmed his prejudices; in Stevenson's it has not.

Stevenson and his colleagues did not discuss any theory of society behind their construct, which probably therefore reflected their own class experiences and prejudices. At the beginning of the century, a raging debate was under way between the hereditarians in the eugenic movement, led by Galton, and the environmentalists who argued that health was a product of the social and political environment. Szreter suggests that the social class classification was part of this argument. While Stevenson's mentor, Newsholme, held environmentalist views, Stevenson's seemed much more eclectic and complex although he probably leaned more towards the environmentalist than hereditarian interpretation. His environmentalist leanings may have acted as a catalyst to producing a social class analysis which reinforced non-hereditarian interpretations. In the event, the social class classification rests on a number of assumptions; that social inequality is an inherent feature of our society; that this can be represented by a single continuous hierarchical scale; that this exists throughout all British society, regardless of place or community; that this scale measures the status of each individual in society; and that current occupation is the most appropriate indicator of this. While the first assumption is undoubtedly true, the others are not. It is not surprising that epidemiologists have attempted to measure those aspects of society which affect behaviour and hence health and ill-health. What is surprising is the banality of the Registrar General's social class classification as a method for doing this. Szreter has concluded that the Registrar General's social class classification is an obsolete pseudo-analytical conceptual framework which, if retained, would be best renamed the 'Crude Inequality Index', but could more usefully be abandoned. By doing this, it would free us from a particular perception, which has now become a self-perpetuating myth, that we live in a society which has an unchanging hierarchy of five grades.

Not only is the classification a value-laden manipulation of the data, but more importantly it is an empiricist construct. The 'classes' devised by Stevenson and his successors are not social classes at all. They are merely groupings of occupations compiled illegitimately with no theoretical basis and have no scientific standing. A common riposte, one employed by Stevenson (1928) himself, is that theory is unnecessary because this crude index works. Theoretical rigour is still considered unnecessary by those who have called for social class data in the United States of America, even although it is anti-intellectual and inhibits progress. Moreover, the classification does not work in that mortality and morbidity statistics analysed by social classes are, at the end of the day, merely weighted means of the rates in their constituent occupations, which do not represent fairly these constituents. There appears no satisfactory answer to what is to be gained by continuing to use it. Perhaps some believe that mortality experience can be changed by changing people's social class. This does not work. Stevenson has shown that. The development more recently of alternative social class classifications, including the ACORN group, the Jarman index, and the Carstairs index, has been an implicit response to the unsatisfactory nature of the Registrar General's. However, none of the single indicator measures based on occupation, housing or education satisfactorily addresses the inherent problem. Composite measures are no more appropriate, and many are worthy examples of the ecological fallacy which transfers relationships which occur in populations to individuals.

Similar criticisms have been levelled against the racial and ethnic classifications used for a long time by North American epidemiologists, and defended using the same empiricist arguments (Buehler et al., 1990). These, or analogous, classifications are increasingly employed and criticised in British research. Critique of the conceptual framework, however, does not seem to diminish the apparent need for researchers to categorise people by race or ethnicity. Even doubts about the very validity of these terms as 'variables' can be overcome on the grounds of expediency, particularly if enough data are collected. Official editorial approval has now been given to a minimum list that is expected of researchers and this includes genetic differences, self-assigned ethnicity, observer-assigned ethnicity, country or area of birth, years in country of residence and religion (Anonymous, 1996). These racist classifications have therefore been lent credibility, and the same kind of justification given for continuing the process that Stevenson and Newsholme used for social class classification at the beginning of the century — with equally banal consequences and potential dangers. The latter are well illustrated by reference to the respected Black report on inequalities in health in which being of a lower social class is equated with being black (DHSS, 1980). This repugnant, though undoubtedly unintentional and thoughtless, example of medical racism by well-meaning individuals was subsequently admitted by Sir Douglas Black (BMA, 1985) himself, and expunged from later published editions of the report.

Empiricism as represented by the work of many modern epidemiologists is sterile and cannot form a satisfactory basis for scientific advance whether the investigation is about social class, race, ethnicity, deprivation, risk factor or any one of the other myriad 'variables' which permeate the literature. It is a misuse of epidemiological techniques and encourages 'Scotch broth' epidemiology in which a number of these variables are added to a pot, stirred around, and sieved to see what is left. This is then presented as if the product was the outcome of careful prior thought and hypotheses. A sustained critique of it can be found in the work of the American sociologist C. Wright Mills (1970). In a chapter entitled 'Abstracted empiricism', he notes that it has a pronounced tendency to confuse the subject under investigation with the methods to be used. The thinness of the results is matched only by the meticulous care in applying elaborate and complex methods, the latter frequently being statistical or epidemiological to give a pseudo-mathematical veneer of legitimacy. The methodology and ease of collection determine the problems and the details are unconvincing of anything worth having convictions about. The extent to which empiricism has a legitimate place in epidemiology is much debated. A detailed Marxist critique of empiricism and other ideologies has been given by Allen (1975).

ECLECTICISM

Many practitioners do not admit to any single ideology or theory we have discussed. They do not see merit in taking sides. Indeed, they see positive merit in not taking sides: they are eclectic, selecting those parts of different theories which seem most appealing to their immediate needs. Not infrequently this leads to syncretism, the co-existence of mutually incompatible theories. In doing so they fail to appreciate that progress depends on their taking sides.

Medical eclecticism reached its apogee in Germany during the Nazi era, during which a concatenation of empiricism, social Darwinism and objectivism combined to produce the horrors of the holocaust. The role of the medical profession, of which more than half belonged to the ruling party, the highest proportion of any profession, has been extensively investigated and reviewed. A long period of racial classification of Jews and others into Aryan and non-Aryan categories resulted in this empiricist approach becoming part of ideology, acceptable and the norm. A strong eugenic movement increasingly concerned itself with the social impact of eugenics and with racial hygiene. This was enthusiastically endorsed by the leading medical authorities of the time. The belief that Jews, the 'feeble minded', socialists, communists, gypsies and others were extra-human combined with these to produce the tragic consequences we all know. The medical profession, far from being a passive observer, and to its everlasting ignominy, was among the cheer leaders.

MATERIALISM IN PRACTICE

The fourth and final paper in the series by Cameron and Jones (1985) attempted to show how a materialist or Marxist analysis addressed a pressing social problem and by sociological analysis could arrive at an understanding of it and of the kind of action needed to prevent illhealth. Since the whole range of human disease was impractical to examine, 'drugs of solace' were chosen as an example.

Drugs of solace were defined as encompassing natural and synthetic products which have been used for the relief of pain and human suffering over the years. They include what are termed hard and soft drugs, sedatives, tranquillisers, stimulants, solvents, tobacco and alcohol. Most societies now adopt a syncretic approach to these substances: on the one hand, most receive official endorsement under various circumstances; on the other society also prohibits their use. Their sale and distribution are legally controlled to greater or lesser degrees. Some can be bought at virtually any time of the day or night, whereas others are only available on prescription. The use of still others, although widely available, is prohibited in some or most societies.

The paper made two propositions: first, that society makes use of these drugs to relieve people of pain and suffering, very often that which is either not brought to the attention of doctors or unrelieved by them; secondly, that the conditions which lead to the need for these drugs, and hence the medical consequences of dependence, addiction, intoxication and organ damage, are twofold. The first of these conditions comprise those where the material causes are clearly understood and direct, and the second in which they act indirectly and through ideology. In the case of alcohol and tobacco, this ideology is the dominant ideology supporting the ruling capitalist class.

These drugs are not diseases; nor is taking them. They are essentially folk remedies for conditions which generally do not find their way into official disease classifications and for which medicine cannot or does not offer help. Rather medicine sees its role as offering to treat their unwanted side effects.

The current epidemiological approach tends to result in counting the numbers of people who are taking these drugs, or treated for their complications, or convicted of offences as a result of taking them. However, as far as the drugs of solace are concerned, the numbers are so great as to involve most of society. Each group therefore constitutes a biased sample for whom that particular drug was the most suitable for them in their circumstances, both social and ideological. People take them to compensate for disharmony between themselves and their environment. Some of this is material such as adverse social circumstances or inappropriate education to prepare them to cope with life crises and some, such as sexual competence, ideological.

Tobacco and alcohol are needed by our society for a number of reasons. First, they console individuals who suffer from adverse conditions our society is unable to ameliorate and for which capitalist society has no programme for achieving. Secondly, from an economic standpoint, they are both an easy source of huge amounts of tax revenue, and also serve to soak up disposable income. Thirdly, by accelerating death in the middle aged and elderly, they save the state large sums of money in social support of various kinds. Fourthly, they provide a need and support for other industries, including the pharmaceutical industry. Finally, they disable people from protest and political activities which might otherwise make government more open to question. Ideology presents these in a favourable light, since no government would dare subscribe to any of these motives.

In any society, different and competing ideologies can co-exist. Ideologies are not fixed; they change according to the prevailing political and social environment. The drugs of solace are a case in point. Ideology has for centuries been extremely favourable to alcohol in most non-Islamic societies but most unfavourable in certain middle eastern and Asian countries. Ideology is universally unfavourable to heroin, cocaine and similar substances; the use of tranquillisers and sedatives when prescribed by doctors is sanctioned by ideology, but not when these drugs are taken without medical approval.

The position with tobacco is rapidly changing and is an example of a victim-led ideological shift. When it was first introduced to England in 1604, it had a bad press; over the centuries this changed until it reached a high point among the Allies during the two World Wars and shortly thereafter. On the other hand, it received the opprobrium of the Nazis during their rule in Germany. Over the last 30 years it has increasingly become clear that tobacco has serious consequences for health, a situation which has arisen because of official medical reports, tragedies such as the King's Cross disaster and the personal experiences of members of the public. Governments are increasingly levying greater burdens of taxation on the product. Greater numbers of non-smokers becoming more insistent of their 'right' to breathe tobacco-free air is putting more pressure on governments to take some action and making smokers feel more and more isolated. At the same time, pressure is being put on government to take some measures against tobacco. The overall effect is a gradual withdrawal of ideological support for tobacco especially in the United States of America and in the United Kingdom. The response of the trans-national tobacco companies is a rear-guard action to defend its position, and the targeting of young people and the developing countries in the hope that their loss of sales in the advanced capitalist countries will be more than compensated by increased profit from elsewhere.

In contrast, a consumer-led ideological shift is occurring with marijuana. Although illegal in most countries, its use especially among the young in North America and Europe has reached such high levels that the state in its authoritative mode, through the police, courts and prison services, can no longer cope. There are parallels between this and the situation during the Prohibition period in the United States of America. As a result, the police increasingly turn a blind eye to its use and the courts become more lenient. In the case of the Netherlands, its use is officially condoned, although disapproved of. In the years ahead, as more and more people use it and hence give it tacit approval, and it becomes a larger industry, it is likely that the tobacco trans-nationals and others will see another potential source of profit. Pressure will then be brought to bear on governments not only to legalise it but sanction its controlled manufacture. Such a situation cannot be far off.

Action against any one drug of solace in isolation is no solution, since the result is merely a shift in use from one to another. Part of the solution is to remove the need for people to take these drugs in the first place. In the case of alcohol in particular, it is difficult to imagine how such a preventive measure is likely to be devised or implemented successfully in the foreseeable future. In any case, it is certainly impossible without a sociological analysis, as is the devising of a strategy to solve the problems it currently creates. Medicine has given too much emphasis in the past to the substance and not enough to the underlying circumstances that make its consumption necessary. Putting effort on the physiological and psychological consequences of the use of alcohol, and the other drugs of solace, to the exclusion of the social circumstances being tackled will not bring about a significant reduction in their use.

A CRITIQUE OF MARXISM IN PUBLIC HEALTH

The political literature in support of and against a Marxist analysis of society is immense. Perhaps the best known recent English language philosopher who has criticised Marxism familiar to those in the public health field is Karl Popper (1966), and this in turn has been subjected to critical appraisal by Cornforth (1968). Marxist critiques are much less common in the general medical literature, although they do appear from time to time (Navarro, 1983), and sometimes Marxist analysis of class is employed by writers who subscribe to piecemeal social engineering (Wright, 1995). They are unusual in the public health literature. One exception appeared in a critical review of the Black report (Strong, 1990). Strong's thesis is that the Black Committee chose just one measure of class, the Registrar General's social class classification, and only one mode of class analysis, that of Marx, and ignored the rest. He then proceeds to make two major criticisms of Marxists, first that they are utopian and secondly that they are economic reductionists. Such views are widespread, although the latter opinion is not shared by Popper (ibid, p.100), who felt that these misinterpreted Marx. Strong's reasoning for the first proposition is that all human progress since Neolithic times has been accompanied by major economic inequality, and he considers it unlikely on current evidence that matters would be any different in some future society. Strong is, of course, correct in discussing the inequality of economic progress up to and including capitalist society. Marx himself puts forward the underlying analysis of this and touches on economic relationships in socialist society in Capital. Both Marx and Engels were well aware of Strong's second proposition and Popper was clearly also aware of their attempts to deal with this criticism. Engels (1890) dealt with the issue in a letter to Bloch, where he wrote that, although the economic ones are ultimately decisive others including political ones and traditions also play a part.

CONSEQUENCES OF LACK OF EXPLICIT THEORY

The Epidemiological Ethos

Strong's claim that Marxism is basically reductionist is an assertion that could readily be levelled against much public health as it is generally practised today. It is one of a number of problems arising as a result of most of its leading exponents' lacking a specific theoretical base. Simple explanations for complex problems are legion in public health literature, 'risk factors', being a good example. The lack of intellectual foundation to risk factors has been highlighted in the past, but they are superficially attractive as they are simple to apply and avoid the need to admit lack of knowledge. They are but one example of the epidemiological ethos, the inappropriate application of techniques derived from the study of epidemics, where the underlying cause or causes are known, to diseases and conditions for which the necessary cause or causes are unknown. Epidemiology's role is to elucidate the sufficient causes once these necessary ones have been established. For example, epidemiology has nothing to offer in elucidating sufficient causes and thus preventive strategies for coronary heart disease as the necessary cause or causes remain unknown. This is not to say that there is total agreement on what constitutes 'cause', since even the most simple examples such as accidents for which both the necessary and sufficient causes are clear can be made complex by taking enquiry to extremes.

The Bureaucratic Ethos

C. Wright Mills (1970) discusses the bureaucratic ethos extensively in writing about the sociological imagination. It is exemplified in public health by a fawning deference to bureaucratic institutions, including health departments, health authorities and their officials. Mills characterises it as the elaboration of concepts, which have nothing to do with any research findings but rather with the legitimisation of the regime and of its changing features. He notes that theory serves as the ideological justification of authority and that research for bureaucratic ends makes the authority more effective and efficient. The bureaucratic ethos has a strong element of personal ambition, or at least the pursuit of a strategy of self-interest, superimposed on an ideology of objectivism.

The Apostatic Ethos

Lack of specific sociological theory has resulted in never-ending introspection and a changing response to the nature of public health, not only in Britain but elsewhere. New movements have produced new names for the discipline, but failure to deliver other than rhetoric has resulted in repeated episodes of disappointment, disillusionment and academic downfall. In the 1970s, British public health evinced a model in which the technique of epidemiology would provide the support for health service management and this managerial role prevailed. It did not last long. When purchasing and providing became the vogue in the 1990s the model changed overnight to a purchaser model to the exclusion of providing, and this without any critical appraisal of why the previous one did not work or was inappropriate. In spite of specific statements to the contrary it is difficult to convince oneself that the movement over the last few years to broaden the membership of the Faculty of Public Health Medicine in Britain is motivated by altruism or a fundamental appreciation of the principles underlying a 'new' role for public health rather than the need to recruit members to stay in business. There appear to be parallels between these events and the rice Christians recruited by Western missionaries in Asia last century. Self-preservation is a powerful human driving force. In the last resort a social explanation of health and ill-health, for which a sociological theory is needed, offers a more powerful model.

The Number-crunching Ethos

This is an extreme form of empiricism which involves a tendency to activity of negligible practical benefit to other people and is generally a by-product of an asocial outlook on life in someone whose job involves the processing of large amounts of data, for which the advent of the computer has been manna from heaven. Sometimes it is manifest in academics with research grants for carrying out 'epidemiological' studies of a similar nature. No epidemiologist would ever own up to such a discreditable ethos for very obvious reasons, and the product of their labour is always elaborately justified and identified with the natural as opposed to the social sciences.

A WAY FORWARD

Concerns about the general direction of public health are not new; neither is the need for principles to underpin its practice. One response to this was an international workshop in Leeds, England in 1993, the outcome of which was the Leeds Declaration (Scott-Samuel, 1994). It brought together a range of individuals from a variety of disciplines within the broad sphere of public health and with widely different ideological perspectives. These individuals were united, however, in the need for public health to re-focus upstream, to move away from individual risks towards social structures and processes from which health and ill-health originate and this was the substance of the first of the ten principles in the declaration. The declaration offers a way forward for public health. Public health practitioners need a theory of society, or sociology, to act as a guide when they apply their collection of techniques which come within the umbrella of epidemiology. Without one, their practice is unscientific or at best a proto-science. Choosing an explicit theory in itself from those that are available will not make for better decisions, make us appear more relevant or guarantee we attain our objectives of promoting the public health, since these will depend on which theory we chose. It will however allow us to make conscious decisions rather than shots in the dark. It will also allow us and others to understand the reasons for these decisions and hopefully avoid some of our mistakes.

In choosing a theory, public health practitioners must be conscious of the strengths and weaknesses of each. We have been quite explicit in declaring our own materialist ethos. In making this choice, we are acutely aware of the disadvantages of being associated with the discredited policies and practices of countries which espoused a Marxist ideology. Nevertheless, we believe that only a materialist theory of society and health offers an internally and externally consistent foundation for fulfilling the public health role of promoting well-being and reducing ill-health.

REFERENCES

Allen V L 1975 Social Analysis: A Marxist Critique and Alternative. The Moor Press, Shipley

Anonymous 1996 Ethnicity, race, and culture: guidelines for research, audit, and publication. British Medical Journal 312: 1094

British Medical Association 1985 Inequalities in health: report of the symposium held on the occasion of the 1985 junior members forum. British Medical Association, London

Buehler J W, Berkelman R L, Stroup D F, Klaucke D N 1990 Authors' response. Public Health Reports 105: 103

Burry J N 1996 The place of Darwin and his theory within history studies. Proceedings of the Royal College of Physicians of Edinburgh 26: 622–8

Cameron D, Jones I G 1982 Theory in community medicine. Community Medicine 4: 3–11

Cameron D, Jones I G 1983 John Snow, the Broad Street pump and modern epidemiology. International Journal of Epidemiology 12: 393–6

Cameron D, Jones I G 1985 An epidemiological and sociological analysis of the use of alcohol, tobacco and other drugs of solace. Community Medicine 7: 18–29

Cornforth M 1968 The Open Philosophy and the Open Society. Lawrence and Wishart, London

Cornell J, Milner P 1996 Is health a matter of choice? Journal of Public Health Medicine 18: 127–8

Department of Health and Social Security 1980 Inequalities in Health. DHSS, London

Engels F 1890. in Karl Marx and Frederick Engels: Selected works in one volume 1968. Lawrence and Wishart, London

Jones I G, Cameron D 1984 Social class analysis – an embarrassment to epidemiology. Community Medicine 6: 37–46

Leete R, Fox J 1977 Registrar General's social classes: origins and uses. Population Trends 8: 1–7

Mackintosh N J 1996 Science struck dumb. Nature 381: 33

Mills C W 1970 The Sociological Imagination. Penguin Books, Harmondsworth

Navarro V 1983 Radicalism, Marxism, and medicine. International Journal of Health Services 13: 179–202

Poor Law Commissioners 1842 Report on an inquiry into the sanitary condition of the labouring population of Great Britain. HMSO, London. Reprinted by Edinburgh University Press 1965

Popper K R 1966 The Open Society and its Enemies. Volume II. The high tide of prophecy: Hegel, Marx, and the aftermath. Routledge and Kegan Paul, London

Registrar General 1913 Seventy-fourth Annual Report of the Registrar-General of births, deaths, and marriages in England and Wales (1911). HMSO, London

Registrar General 1923 Supplement to the 75th Annual Report of the Registrar General for England and Wales. Part IV. Mortality of men in certain occupations in the three years 1910, 1911, and 1912. HMSO, London

Scott-Samuel A 1994 New responses in research and practice. Health Education Journal 53: 113–15

Stevenson T H C 1923 The social distribution of mortality from different causes in England and Wales, 1910–12. Biometrika 15: 382–400

Stevenson T H C 1928 The vital statistics of wealth and poverty. Journal of the Royal Statistical Society 91: 207–20

Strong P M 1990 Black on class and mortality: theory, method and history. Journal of Public Health Medicine 12: 168–80

Szreter S R S 1984 The genesis of the Registrar-General's social classification of occupations. British Journal of Sociology 35: 522–46

Wright E O 1995 The class analysis of poverty. International Journal of Health Services 25: 85–100

6. Inequalities in Health: What is happening and what can be done?

George Davey Smith and Yoav Ben-Shlomo

INTRODUCTION

Mortality differentials according to socio-economic group have long been recognised in the UK. In 1845, Engels reproduced such data, using both area-based and individual indicators of socio-economic status (Table 6.1) (Engels, 1845). Engels went on to quote from the Report on the Sanitary Conditions of the Working Class:

In Liverpool in 1840 the average life-span of the upper classes, gentry, professional men, etc, was thirty-five years; that of the business men and better-placed handicraftsmen, twenty-two years; and that of the operatives, day-labourers, and serviceable class in general, but fifteen years.

Socio-economic differentials in mortality appear to have persisted from the time of Engels' description of early Victorian conditions until the present day (Davey Smith *et al.*,1990a; 1992; Davey Smith & Morris, 1994). The best longitudinal series of such data available internationally comes from statistics on social class mortality differences produced around each British census. Figure 6.1 presents mortality rates for middle-aged men from the years around the 1921

Table 6.1 Mortality ratios (number of living people for each death) in Chorlton-on-Medlock, Manchester

Class of street	Class of house		
	1st	2nd	3rd
1st	51/1	45/1	36/1
2nd	55/1	38/1	35/1
3rd	-*	35/1	25/1

* no data.
Source: Engels, 1845.

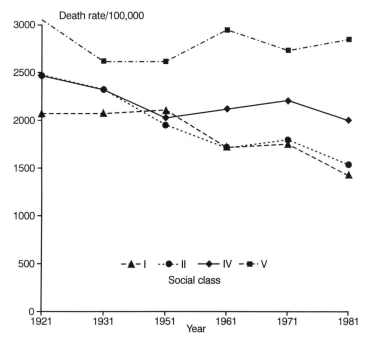

Fig.6.1 Death rates per 100,000 men aged 55–64 in England and Wales, 1921–1981. (Source: Blane *et al.*, 1997.)

census to the years around the 1981 census. Dramatic declines in mortality are seen for social class I and II, while for social class IV and V small and inconsistent decreases in mortality are seen (Blane *et al.*, 1997). Increases in both the relative and absolute differentials in mortality between the social class groups have occurred since the early 1950s (Pamuk, 1985); a pattern which recent data demonstrate has continued throughout the 1980s (Harding, 1995; Drever *et al.*, 1996). Recent analysis for the years arounds the 1991 census (Fig. 6.2) demonstrate substantial social class differences in all cause mortality for men; whilst data for women have yet to appear. For males of working ages, the relative differentials in mortality for all-causes, stroke, ischaemic heart disease, lung cancer and suicide have continued to increase (Drever *et al.*, 1996). While a decline in mortality rate for social class V men occurred between 1981 and 1991, mortality in 1991 is still higher than in 1971 for this group.

Morbidity data according to social position are more difficult to locate than mortality data. A series of recent studies has demonstrated that common forms of morbidity demonstrate the same socio-eco-

England and Wales: Male all-cause mortality 1991–1993

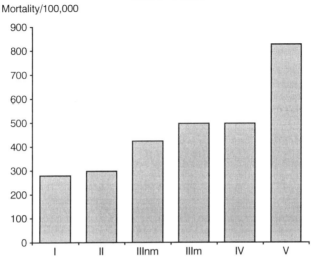

Fig. 6.2   Death rates per 100,000 men aged 20–64 according to social class, 1992–1993. (Source: Drever *et al.*, 1996.)

nomic patterning as does mortality and limiting long-term illness (Marmot *et al.*, 1991; Eachus *et al.*, 1996). Table 6.2 displays the differing prevalences of various chronic conditions according to the socio-economic characteristics of area of residence in a sample of more than 20,000 men and women in Somerset and Avon. The introduction of a question regarding 'limiting long-term illness' in the 1991 census has allowed the strong and consistent associations of chronic morbidity with deprivation to be demonstrated (Bentham *et al.*, 1995). Reliable data on trends in socio-economic differentials in morbidity from particular causes are not available, however.

INVESTIGATING THE ORIGINS OF SOCIO-ECONOMIC DIFFERENTIALS IN HEALTH

Several reviews of the contribution of different sets of factors to socio-economic differentials in health have appeared recently (Whitehead, 1992; Davey Smith *et al.*, 1994a; Marmot *et al.*, 1995). They have extensively considered the degree to which observed inequalities in health may be artefactual, that is, produced by the ways in which data are collected and analysed. Such processes

Table 6.2 Age standardised prevalence per 100 of self-reported diseases by deprivation category

	1st fifth	2nd fifth	3rd fifth	4th fifth	5th fifth	P value
Men						
Musculoskeletal diseases	14.1	15.1	16.1	16.1	17.7	<0.001
Angina	4.4	5.5	5.5	5.5	6.9	<0.001
Myocardial infarction	3.2	3.7	4.0	4.5	4.8	<0.001
Asthma	5.6	6.1	6.2	6.4	6.4	0.18
Bronchitis	5.2	6.3	7.3	7.7	9.1	<0.001
Depression	3.9	4.8	5.9	6.2	6.9	<0.001
Stroke	2.0	1.8	1.3	2.3	2.6	0.03
Diabetes	2.4	2.5	3.7	2.7	2.1	0.83
Diabetic eye disease	0.5	0.6	0.9	1.0	0.7	0.05
Women						
Musculoskeletal diseases	27.3	28.6	30.6	30.5	34.5	<0.001
Angina	3.8	4.4	4.6	4.4	5.8	<0.002
Myocardial infarction	1.5	1.9	1.7	1.8	2.5	0.03
Asthma	6.4	6.2	7.5	7.0	9.8	<0.001
Bronchitis	7.5	8.1	9.0	10.2	13.2	<0.001
Depression	10.1	10.5	11.4	12.5	12.7	<0.001
Stroke	1.6	2.0	2.1	2.2	2.4	0.04
Diabetes	2.6	2.4	2.1	2.1	2.4	0.56
Diabetic eye disease	0.6	0.5	0.6	0.7	1.5	<0.001

Source: Eachus *et al.*, 1996.

appear, if anything, to lead to under-estimation, rather than over-estimation, of the magnitude of health inequalities. This relates both to measurement of socio-economic position and the measurement of health. Conventional measures of socio-economic position suffer from a lack of discriminatory power and the use of enriched indicators leads to the demonstration of greater mortality and morbidity gradients (Davey Smith *et al.*, 1994a). Differences in the way in which social groups report ill-health may also dilute associations between social position and serious morbidity (Mackenbach *et al.*, 1996; Elstad, 1996). The notion that health determines social position through health-related social mobility, rather than poor health being produced by adverse socio-economic circumstances, is also not supported in any simple way by the available data (Blane *et al.*, 1993).

Several studies have investigated the contribution of particular health-related behaviours and physiological risk factors to mortality differentials. In the first Whitehall study, considerable differences in mortality risk were demonstrated according to two socio-economic indicators: employment grade in the civil service and car ownership (Fig. 6.3) (Davey Smith *et al.*, 1990b). While the lower grade and non-car owning civil servants were more likely to smoke than the higher grade and car owning ones, the pattern of mortality differentials was identical among men who had never smoked (Fig. 6.4) (Davey Smith & Shipley 1991; Davey Smith *et al.*, 1994a).

Cholesterol levels were higher among high rather than low grade civil servants in the late 1960s, when this study was established. Differences in cholesterol levels could not, therefore, account for the higher rates of coronary heart disease among the lower grade employees. This can be taken to suggest that differences in dietary fat intake between grades in this cohort were not responsible for the

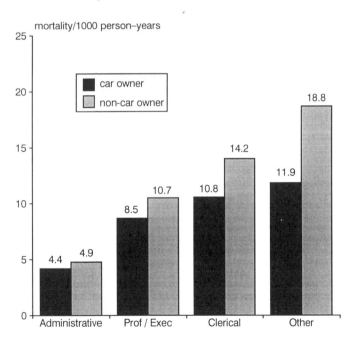

Fig. 6.3   Mortality by employment grade and car ownership in the Whitehall study. (Source: Davey Smith *et al.*, 1990b.)

mortality/1000 person–years

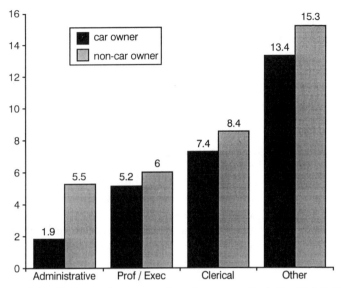

Fig. 6.4 Mortality by employment grade and car ownership in the Whitehall study among men who had never smoked. (Source: Davey Smith *et al.*, 1990b.)

coronary heart disease mortality differentials. Indeed, simultaneous consideration of a range of risk factors (including smoking, blood pressure, cholesterol levels and prevalent cardio-respiratory disease) failed to account for the grade differences in cardiovascular and non-cardiovascular mortality (Davey Smith *et al.*, 1990b).

Similar findings have emerged from a study in the West of Scotland established around the same time as the first Whitehall study (Davey Smith *et al.*, 1994b; 1997). Large differentials in cardiovascular disease mortality according to both educational attainment and social class existed at a time when blood cholesterol levels were highest in those with the most education and in the professional and managerial classes. Adjustments for a wide range of risk factors failed to explain the considerable mortality differentials from major causes of death in this study.

As a result of findings suggesting that conventional risk factors could not explain socio-economic differentials in health, the Whitehall II cohort was established in 1985 to investigate additional factors which might contribute to the social gradients (Marmot *et al.*,

1991). The Whitehall II study found differentials in prevalent ECG abnormalities in both sexes at baseline, which paralleled the findings in the original cohort. In this more recent study, mean total cholesterol levels again appeared not to contribute to the occupational gradient in coronary heart disease risk, as in both sexes the mean cholesterol level at baseline was similar in each grade. Concentrations of serum apolipoprotein AI, the main structural protein of HDL cholesterol, did show an association with grade (Brunner *et al.*, 1993) and suggested that characteristic disturbances of metabolism associated with lower occupational status were potentially identifiable.

Central, or male-type, obesity, which has long been recognised as a factor predisposing to diabetes and coronary disease (Vague 1956), is in both sexes more prevalent amongst the lower grade civil servants. The related components of the metabolic, or insulin resistance syndrome, of elevated triglycerides and a higher prevalence of impaired glucose tolerance are also found more commonly among the lower grade civil servants (Davey Smith and Brunner, 1997).

Low level of control over the nature of one's work, i.e. little ability to decide what one does, and when, has emerged as a potential coronary heart disease risk factor. In the Whitehall II study, low level of job control is associated with an increased risk of coronary heart disease among both men and women, whether measured by self-reports or by external assessments of job characteristics (Bosma *et al.*, 1997). It is, however, difficult to separate low control over work from other aspects of the socio-economic environment (Carroll *et al.*, 1996). Indeed certain aspects of work relations may be considered a fundamental complement of social stratification in capitalist economies (Braverman, 1974).

A study of Finnish men constitutes the most detailed prospective investigation of factors contributing to the socio-economic gradient in cardiovascular mortality undertaken to date (Lynch *et al.*, 1996). The risk of all-cause and cardiovascular disease mortality across quintiles of adulthood income showed two- to threefold differences. It was possible to adjust for 22 risk factors: plasma fibrinogen, serum HDL cholesterol, serum apolipoprotein B, blood leukocytes, serum copper, mercury in hair, serum ferritin, blood haemoglobin, serum triglycerides, systolic blood pressure, body mass index, height, cardio-respiratory fitness, cigarette smoking, alcohol consumption, leisure time physical activity, depression, hopelessness, cynical hostility, participation in organisations, quality of social support and marital status (Lynch *et al.*, 1996). On adjustment for all these factors, the association between social position and cardiovascular disease mortality was greatly attenuated, while the associations between social positions and all (fatal and non-fatal) coronary heart disease (CHD) incidence remained substantial. As the authors acknowledge, it is difficult to interpret such analyses, for several reasons. First, some of the factors adjusted for may be markers of disease presence (e.g. blood leukocytes, fibrinogen), and statistical adjustment for these could, in essence, be adjusting for the presence of cardiovascular disease, which is itself produced by social factors. The reduction in relative risks in the lower income groups which occurs on adjustment for these factors cannot be taken as demonstrating the 'explanation' of why the social distribution of cardiovascular mortality exists. Secondly, some factors, e.g. height, body mass index, serum triglycerides, may be the outcome of socio-economic processes, which act in early life. Adjusting for these factors similarly fails to account for the reasons for the social distribution in cardiovascular mortality, since it automatically leads to questions as to how childhood social conditions may influence growth, insulin resistance syndrome and thus coronary disease risk. Finally, the reasons for the social distribution of certain behaviour, e.g. smoking and exercise, itself should become a target for explanation (Davey Smith & Morris 1994).

LIFECOURSE INFLUENCES ON HEALTH INEQUALITIES

Until recently, debates regarding inequalities in health generally related to the relationship between socio-economic circumstances in adulthood and poor health. There has recently been a revival of interest in the effects of poor social circumstances in early life on health in adulthood (Kuh & Davey Smith, 1993). The UK Department of Health report *Variations in Health* (Department of Health, 1995) has recognised the importance of a lifecourse perspective on inequalities in health. It concludes that it

is likely that cumulative differential lifetime exposure to health-damaging or health-promoting physical and social environments is the main explanation for observed variations in health and life expectancy.

Few empirical data regarding such cumulative effects exist, however. In a cohort study in which men have been followed for over 20 years in the west of Scotland (Davey Smith *et al.*, 1997) it was possible to relate mortality experience to the social class of the fathers of the study participants; to the social class of their first occupation on entering the labour market; and to the social class of their occupation at the time of screening, when aged 35–64. In Table 6.3 it is demonstrated that cumulative social class, together with indicators of socio-economic position at the time of screening are strongly associated with mortality risk. When social class locations at different periods of the lifecourse are related to mortality from specific causes, it is seen that the social class of the fathers of the men and their own social class at the time of screening independently contribute to all-cause mortality (Table 6.4). This suggests that there are some long-lasting influences of socio-economic circumstances in childhood on mortality in adulthood. With respect to particular causes of death, childhood socio-economic conditions have particular importance for cardiovascular disease, but are related less strongly to cancer and other mortality. The suggestion that mortality risk reflects the accumulation of environmental insults or the cumulative effects of unfavourable behavioural or psychological factors which progressively increase susceptibility to disease (Jones, 1956; Alter & Riley, 1989) is supported by a study based on record linkage of the 1960, 1970 and 1980 census records for Norway, in which particularly high mortality risks are seen among men who obtain limited education and then go on to work in manual occupations and live in poor housing (Salhi et al., 1995). Similar findings have come from the US national longitudinal study of older men (Mare, 1990). The particular dependence of cardiovascular disease risk on childhood socio-economic circumstances in comparison to

Table 6.3 All cause mortality by cumulative social class, car driving, and deprivation category of area of residence. Values are age adjusted relative rates (95% confidence intervals)

	Cumulative social class			
	All three non-manual	Two non-manual one manual	Two manual, one non manual	All three manual
Regular car driver:				
Yes	1	1.28 (1.01 to 1.63)	1.36 (1.08 to 1.73)	1.57 (1.27 to 1.95)
No	1.22 (0.91 to 1.64)	1.52 (1.19 to 1.95)	1.76 (1.40 to 2.21)	2.00 (1.64 to 2.44)
Deprivation category of area of residence				
1–4	1	1.25 (1.01 to 1.56)	1.37 (1.09 to 1.72)	1.70 (1.39 to 2.09)
5–7	1.06 (0.74 to 1.52)	1.41 (1.10 to 1.82)	1.54 (1.25 to 1.90)	1.74 (1.45 to 2.09)

Table 6.4 Mortality by social class at three different stages of life, manual versus non-manaual relative rates

	Father's social class	First social class	Current social class
All causes			
Individual	1.44 (1.27 to 1.64)	1.29 (1.16 to 1.43)	1.40 (1.27 to 1.55)
Simultaneous	1.28 (1.11 to 1.47)	1.01 (0.89 to 1.16)	1.29 (1.14 to 1.47)
Cardiovascular causes			
Individual	1.58 (1.32 to 1.89)	1.35 (1.16 to 1.56)	1.38 (1.13 to 1.61)
Simultaneous	1.41 (1.15 to 1.72)	1.08 (0.90 to 1.30)	1.20 (1.01 to 1.43)
Cancer			
Individual	1.26 (1.02 to 1.56)	1.25 (1.04 to 1.50)	1.35 (1.13 to 1.61)
Simultaneous	1.11 (0.87 to 1.41)	1.04 (0.82 to 1.31)	1.28 (1.03 to 1.60)
Non-cardiovascular, non-cancer causes			
Individual	1.45 (1.07 to 1.98)	1.18 (0.92 to 1.53)	1.59 (1.24 to 2.03)
Simultaneous	1.28 (0.91 to 1.80)	0.80 (0.58 to 1.10)	1.67 (1.22 to 2.28)

Values are age-adjusted relative rates (95% confidence intervals), with individual and simultaneous adjustment for each social class indicator.

other causes of death has been observed in area-based studies from Finland (Valkonen, 1987; Koskinen, 1994).

Of particular current research interest are the long-term effects of development during foetal and early infant life on disease risk in adulthood. A series of ecological and prospective studies have demonstrated that birthweight and weight at one year of age are inversely related to cardiovascular disease risk, diabetes risk and blood pressure in later life (Barker, 1995). While it is difficult to separate out the effects of such early life exposures from later experiences (Ben-Shlomo & Davey Smith, 1991; Bartley et al., 1994), these findings are strongly suggestive of important persisting influences from early life into adulthood. In a study from South Wales, men with low birthweight were at a particularly elevated risk of coronary heart disease if they became obese in adulthood (Frankel et al., 1996) (Fig. 6.5). Thus the socially patterned exposure of suboptimal intrauterine development, indexed by low birthweight, interacts with the socially patterned exposure of obesity in adulthood to generate elevated disease risk.

Less research has been carried out recently on the effects of childhood nutrition on later disease, although earlier this century it was considered unproblematically obvious that such effects did exist (Davey Smith & Kuh, 1996). Preliminary data are now available from a mortality follow-up of the children included in surveys

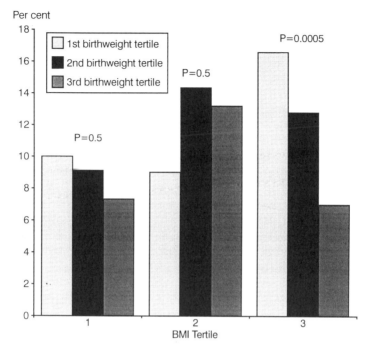

Fig. 6.5   Coronary heart disease incidence by birthweight and body mass index in the Caerphilly study. (Source: Frankel *et al.*, 1996.)

of poverty, nutrition and child health carried out under the auspices of Lord John Boyd Orr in the immediate pre-Second World War period (Rowett Research Institute, 1955). At the time this survey was carried out, it was recognised by one of the investigators that leg length was a particularly good indicator of childhood socio-economic and nutritional circumstances:

When the Carnegie UK Dietary and Clinical Survey was planned at the Rowett Research Institute in 1937, cristal height as a measure of leg length was included in the measurements... it was found that cristal height was consistently better than total height for indicating expenditure group... we find the longer-legged children suffered less bronchitis than the short at all ages. Since there is neither complicating immunity mechanism nor specific cure for bronchitis, we might argue that constitution built up when the complete harmonious pattern of growth is unfolded is, in some way, superior to that associated with inhibition of growth, however slight (Leitch, 1951).

A re-analysis of these data clearly demonstrates this to be the case as age-standardised indicators of total height, leg length and trunk length reveal differential associations with nutritional and socio-economic factors (Gunnell *et al.*, 1996) (Table 6.5). In particular, it is noticeable that the negative correlations between overcrowding and social class of head of household (scored from 1 for professional groups to 5 for unskilled manual workers) are considerably stronger for leg length than for trunk length, while the positive correlations between weighted per capita food expenditure and relative family per capita calorie consumption are similarly stronger for leg length than trunk length. Results for females are similar to those in males.

Leg length in childhood is associated with mortality over the subsequent 60 years (Table 6.6). These data suggest that there may be important long-term consequences of childhood nutrition on health in later life. They do not, however, paint a one-sided view of rapid growth in childhood. In line with evidence from animal studies and some epidemiological findings (Tannenbaum, 1947; Albanes *et al.*, 1988), cancer risk may be increased by greater calorie intake and growth in early life. Thus reductions in cardiovascular disease mortality in response to socio-economic and nutritional conditions which encourage growth in childhood may, in part, be counter-balanced by increases in cancer mortality. Studies which obtain data over the lifecourse of participants are required to untangle the relative contributions of factors acting at different stages of life (and the importance of interactions between such factors across the life course) to further understand their role in generating disease risk in adulthood.

Table 6.5 Pearson's correlation coefficients between anthropometry, childhood dietary and socio-economic variables and adult SES (males)

Anthropometric, dietary or socio-economic index (n)	'z' score for height	'z' score for leg length	'z' score for trunk length
Birth order (1397)	−0.14*	−0.14*	−0.06*
No. of children (1394)	−0.25*	−0.24*	−0.14*
Weighted per capita food expenditure (1394)	0.31*	0.33*	0.14*
Social class of head of household (1287)	−0.18*	−0.21*	−0.05
Overcrowding (1220)	−0.19*	−0.20*	−0.08*
Relative family per capita calorie consumption (1394)	0.23*	0.26*	0.08*

Source: Gunnell *et al.*, 1996.
* $P < 0.05$.

Table 6.6 Leg length and mortality: Carnegie survey follow-up

Quintile	CHD mortality Fully adjusted relative risk (*95% CI)	Cancer mortality Fully adjusted relative risk (*95% CI)
Males		
1 (shortest)	2.8 (1.1,6.9)	0.4 (0.1,1.1)
2	2.5 (1.0,6.0)	0.4 (0.2,1.1)
3	2.2 (0.9,5.2)	0.6 (0.2,1.5)
4	2.5 (1.1,5.7)	0.8 (0.4,1.8)
5 (tallest)	1.0	1.0
Linear trend test	P=0.09	P=0.06
Females		
1 (shortest)	4.2 (0.8,22.2)	1.0 (0.4,2.3)
2	3.5 (0.7,17.8)	1.1 (0.5,2.4)
3	1.9 (0.3,10.6)	1.0 (0.4,2.2)
4	0.9 (0.1,6.6)	0.8 (0.4,2.0)
5 (tallest)	1.0	1.0
Linear trend test	P=0.006	P=0.77

* Adjusted for age and indices of childhood and adult socio-economic circumstances, calorie consumption and birth order.

Source: Gunnell et al., 1996.

HEALTH–RELATED BEHAVIOURS: ARE THEY LIFESTYLE CHOICES?

Writing in 1845, Engels considered that nutritional deficiencies contributed to the poor health of the labouring classes. Rather than take this to indicate poor health-related behaviours amongst this deprived group, he realised that the dependence of dietary adequacy upon financial wherewithal was clear.

The better paid workers, especially those in whose families every member is able to earn something, have good food as long as this state of things lasts; meat daily and bacon and cheese for supper. Where wages are less, meat is used only two or three times a week, and the proportion of bread and potatoes increases. Descending gradually, we find the animal food reduced to a small piece of bacon cut up with the potatoes; lower still, even this disappears, and there remain only bread, cheese, porridge, and potatoes, until on the lowest rung of the ladder, among the Irish, potatoes form the sole food.

Engels recognised that the financial disadvantages of the poor were compounded by other social factors in determining their poor diet.

The payment of wages on Saturday evening meant that workers could only buy their food after the middle class had been given first choice during Saturday morning. When the workers reached the market,

the best has vanished, and, if it was still there, they would probably not be able to buy it. The potatoes which the workers buy are usually poor, the vegetables wilted, the cheese old and of poor quality, the bacon rancid, the meat lean, tough, taken from old, often diseased, cattle, or such as have died a natural death, and not fresh even then, often half decayed.

The working classes were also more liable to be sold adulterated food, because while the rich developed sensitive palates through habitual good eating and could detect adulteration, the poor had little opportunity to cultivate their taste and were unable to detect adulteration. They also had to deal with small retailers who could not sell

even the same quality of goods so cheaply as the largest retailers, because of their small capital and the large proportional expenses of their business,... [and] must knowingly or unknowingly buy adulterated goods in order to sell at the lower prices required, and to meet the competition of the others.

The capitalist class, naturally, failed to acknowledge the poor health generated by the inadequate diet of the working class. Indeed, the philosopher of industrialisation, Andrew Ure, was quoted by Engels as suggesting that the workers pampered themselves into nervous ailments 'by a diet too rich and exciting for their indoor employments'.

Several studies have demonstrated that Engels' conclusions remain applicable today: those least able to purchase a healthy diet, due to financial constraints, are those most likely to be disadvantaged with regard to access to healthy micronutrient-dense food. Thus a shopping basket survey in Glasgow demonstrated that households in a less economically favoured area paid more for a healthy basket of food than households in a more favoured area, while there was no difference in the cost of an unhealthy basket of food. It was also noted that several items of the healthy food basket were simply not available in the less favoured area (Sooman et al., 1993). A similar survey was carried out in London in 1988 and repeated in 1995. At both times, healthy food was more expensive in the deprived area while unhealthy food was slightly cheaper in the deprived area (Lobstein, 1995). This study suggested that the situation for those living in the deprived area had become relatively worse between 1988 and 1995.

Poorer families have been disadvantaged by changes in food retailing. Between 1980 and 1992, the number of food retail outlets decreased by 35% (Department of Health, 1996). This reflects a decline in the number of small grocery retailers and specialist shops, including butchers and greengrocers, and an increase in large supermarkets. Such large retailers tend to be based outside of towns and customers require transport to them. The low rate of car ownership among poorer households makes it difficult for them to utilise these generally cheaper outlets. In essence, the transfer of food retailing from smaller local retailers to large out-of-town superstores represents a transfer of costs from the food wholesaler, who is required to transport food to fewer outlets, to the customer, who must travel further to purchase food. This transfer represents a disproportionate burden to poorer households and contributes to widening inequalities in material circumstances.

Low income households, residing in less affluent areas, are disadvantaged in other ways with respect to food, diet and nutrition. Such households may especially value the social resource represented by the personal nature of local shopping more, given fewer alternative social opportunities. Shopping can become a demoralising experience for those whose choice is constrained by a lack of income (Dowler, 1996). The costs of cooking and of stocking essential items required for food preparation represent additional expenditure which may not be available in less well-off households. Thus the use of convenience foods or items such as sandwiches which require no cooking is encouraged.

In a detailed ethnographic study of the social organisation of nutritional inequities Travers (1996) concluded that

The public discourse most consistent with the findings and experience of this research was apparently informed by an individualistic ideology. Individualism assumes that the current social system provides sufficient and equal opportunity for individuals to move within the social system according to their abilities. Within this ideological construct, poverty results from the individual's failure to seize the opportunity or to work sufficiently hard within the current social structure; it is not a reflection of inadequacies and inequities within that social order.

This need not go unchallenged, however. The women in Travers' study were aware that inequitable pricing policies existed, such that the more expensive food stores are located in the inner-city, closer to the areas of residence of socially and economically disadvantaged households. The women initiated a letter-writing campaign to supermarket managers which resulted in a reduction in the pricing differentials between inner-city and suburban stores.

Other health-related behaviours — such as smoking, leisure time physical activity and excessive alcohol consumption — have been shown to be constrained by the material and psychosocial conditions of life in similar ways to diet (e.g. Cameron & Jones, 1985; Graham, 1988). The need for health promotion approaches, which recognise that such practices are not simple lifestyle choices, are required if the components of the overall pattern of health inequalities which are produced by differential adoption of such behaviours are to be addressed.

INFLUENCES OUTSIDE THE INDIVIDUAL — THE IMPORTANCE OF RESIDENTIAL AREA

It is difficult to define the concept of 'community' and this varies depending on the discipline or theorist (for a detailed review, see Patrick & Wickizer, 1995). However, independent of the particular theoretical framework, there is now a growing body of research which demonstrates that characteristics of areas and communities, as well as individuals, have an impact on health. Many previous ecological studies have shown the strong relationships between area deprivation and mortality (Centerwell, 1984; Carstairs & Morris, 1991). Some have suggested that these relationships simply reflect an increased mortality risk for individuals of lower socio-economic status who reside in such areas and do not reflect any additional area effect (Sloggett & Joshi, 1994). However, this conflicts with findings from other studies. The Alameda county study examined the nine-year mortality rates of residents in Oakland, California. Those subjects living in a federally designated poverty area had around 70% higher all cause mortality (Haan et al., 1987). This persisted after adjustment for a wide array of potentially confounding variables, including individual socio-economic position, health practices, social networks and psychological factors.

The development of multi-level modelling techniques now allow more formal empirical testing of area or 'contextual' effects. Results confirm that area characteristics such as deprivation, enable better prediction of physiological measures such as lung function (Jones & Duncan, 1995), long-term illness (Shouls et al., 1996) and suicide (Congdon, 1996), than does the use of individual risk factors alone. For example evidence from a recent multi-level analysis of data from the Scottish Heart Health Study illustrates the relative importance of area effects (Hart et al., 1997). This study was set up, in part, to examine geographical variations in cardiovascular disease risk factors. Significant area effects were found for diastolic blood pressure, cholesterol, and alcohol consumption, although not for smoking, after individual characteristics had been taken into account.

The magnitude of the area effects were, however, relatively small compared to the effect of the individual factors. In general, developmental and other lifecourse experiences or exposures may act more directly at an individual level and have a greater impact than do indirect contextual effects, which must be mediated through other pathways. However, the above studies have simply modelled the effect of current area of residence and have therefore assumed both non-migration as well as the temporal constancy of area effects. If full residential histories were available on subjects and both temporal as well as geographical effects were modelled, it is likely that the proportion of variance explained by area would be greater.

INFLUENCES OUTSIDE THE INDIVIDUAL — THE IMPORTANCE OF COMMUNITY COHESIVENESS

Valuable epidemiological insights can sometimes be gained through 'natural experiments'. One such example is the so-called 'Roseto-effect'. In the 1960s, it was noted that the town of Roseto, Pennsylvania, which contained an Italian American community, had a strikingly low rate of CHD mortality compared to several neighbouring communities with similar socio-economic characteristics. Investigation ruled the possible role of differential medical services or confounding by conventional risk factors such as smoking. However, it was clear that this close immigrant community had a particularly stable social structure, strong family cohesion and provided a supportive environment. Amongst the younger generation acculturation towards aspects of the generic US experience was evident and hence it was hypothesised that breakdown of traditional values would be accompanied by an increase in mortality. Recent temporal data provide support for this hypothesis. Over a 40-year period, the protective effect of residing in Roseto has disappeared, so that mortality from CHD is now no different from its neighbours (Egolf et al., 1992). It is unlikely that the original low rate of CHD mortality in this community can be explained by any simple genetic model, as this would not explain the rapid subsequent rapid convergence in mortality experience. It, however, only provides indirect evidence on the role of community solidarity.

More general attitudes to the local area and community of residence have been found to be related to measures of anxiety and health. In a Scottish study an area assessment score based on residents' opinions on amenities, problems with the area, poor reputation, neighbourliness, fear of crime, and area satisfaction significantly predicted both anxiety and self-assessed health after adjustment for individual socio-economic status (Sooman & Macintyre, 1995).

It is difficult to know exactly what sort of policies would enhance local community cohesion and satisfaction. Local empowerment is one method which forms an underlying principle behind the 'Healthy Cities' movement (Ashton, 1992). While engaging all the population is a difficult endeavour, measuring and promoting 'civic' communities is possible (Putnam et al., 1993). A socio-political study in Italy set out to understand why local regional governments in the north of Italy were more responsive to local needs than those based in the south. To measure the degree of local 'civicness', community participation in local elections, football matches attendance, membership of clubs and readership of local papers were used as measures of an engaged community. Not surprisingly, areas with more civic engagement also had more responsive institutional structures, although it was not clear that this was directly as a result of local involvement. A re-analysis of these data show that enhanced community participation was associated with lower rates of infant mortality (Hertzman, 1996). It was not, however, associated with premature mortality in middle-aged men, highlighting either the inadequacies of this measure or its more complex inter-relationship with individual-based characteristics.

It is interesting that politicians of all complexions tend to advocate decentralisation and communitarianism, though this usually remains at a rhetorical level rather than contributing to the provision of infrastructure and financial support to enable local communities to experience a real sense of empowerment. The latter approach may, however, both enhance the democratic process and have a beneficial impact on health variations.

Education and health

Many studies have shown a clear linear relationship between educational achievement and mortality from a wide variety of conditions (Tyroler et al., 1993; Diez-Roux et al., 1995). American studies often use education as a proxy marker of socio-economic status instead of income or occupation. It is clear that both education and socio-economic status are usually closely related as occupation and hence income is often determined by educational achievement. However the socio-cultural implications of each measure may have a different meaning, for example, in the ARIC study, white men showed a bigger social differential for prevalent CHD by education (odds ratio 3.8) whilst, for black men, income was a better discriminator (odds ratio 3.4) (Diez-Roux *et al.*, 1995). Education may directly influence knowledge about health-protective behaviours, accessing of health services and psychosocial mechanisms such as engagement in social networks and the ability to cope with life stressors. This may explain why some studies find an independent effect of education after adjustment for either income (Elo & Preston, 1996) or other markers of socio-economic status (Holme *et al.*, 1980). The most detailed study of this issue in the UK (Davey Smith *et al.*, 1994b) finds little residual influence of education after taking adult occupation into account, however, indicating that education may influence health through the better opportunities it creates with respect to the type of employment people get, the income they earn, the living conditions they can afford and the area of residence they can live in.

There is evidence that educational interventions targeted at high risk populations may have long-term benefits (Hertzman & Wiens, 1996), although the outcomes for such studies have not usually been interested in or collected specific health outcome measures. One such example is the Perry Preschool study, which was a trial comparing children allocated to either preschool or no preschool interventions. At age 27, those allocated to the active intervention were more likely to be earning more money, be a home-owner, a high school graduate, and less likely to have had contact with social services or have had five or more arrests. Evidence exists that intervention programmes in infancy, preschool and school-age children can have positive impacts on cognitive development, social-emotional development, and coping skills (Hertzman & Wiens, 1996). Several studies have indicated that benefits are not restricted to the school environment but also result in more positive self-perception and family functioning (Hertzman & Wiens, 1996). It is clear that, in some cases, with appropriate re-enforcement, such changes in self-attitude can produce dramatic alterations to an individual's life trajectory, both in terms of occupation, psychosocial functioning, adult health behaviours and risk of subsequent disease.

THE ROLE OF MEDICAL AND HEALTH-RELATED INTERVENTIONS IN REDUCING INEQUALITIES

A recent Department of Health commissioned review examined all studies with an experimental design that targeted poorer sections of the population in order to reduce inequalities in health (Arblaster *et al.*, 1995). From a large number of original papers, only 94 studies could be identified that met the inclusion criteria, and many were of dubious methodological quality. The characteristics that were found to be associated with greater success were (a) needs assessment and community commitment prior to the intervention, (b) intensive, multi-disciplinary, multi-faceted, interventions delivered in a variety of settings, and (c) face-to-face, culturally appropriate interventions delivered by an appropriate agent with sufficient training. The authors concluded that

It is important that strategies developed to reduce inequalities are not assumed to be having a positive impact simply because the aim is 'progressive' and so rigorous evaluations of promising interventions are important.

The apparent paucity of evidence demonstrating the success of health service interventions in reducing inequalities has led some to take an overly nihilistic view of the possible contribution of such interventions (Foster, 1996). Whilst it is generally accepted that medical care has made only a limited contribution to the improvements in mortality rates seen over this century (McKeown *et al.*, 1975; Mackenbach *et al.*, 1990), there is now much evidence on the effectiveness of certain medical interventions in reducing mortality and morbidity and improving quality of life. For example, it is estimated that medical services in general may add around 5 years towards life expectancy (Bunker *et al.*, 1995).

More specifically, around 3.5% of the decline in CHD mortality in the USA up until the early 1980s could be associated with the impact of coronary artery bypass grafting (Goldman & Cook, 1984), although this may now be substantially altered given developments in this field. Extending care to include all types of cardiac surgery, medical treatments and coronary care units, it is estimated that life expectancy may have been prolonged by an additional 1.2 years at a population level, as well as resulting in a substantial improvement in quality of life (Bunker *et al.*, 1995). These estimates must be treated with some caution, but do make the point that the role of medical interventions may be appreciable. Assuming that these benefits apply equally across the socio-economic spectrum, and that all sections of society access them equitably (see below), then they may play a role in reducing inequalities in mortality for at least some diseases. On the other hand, they could also contribute to the generation of inequalities in health. A suggestion of this is given by the data in Table 6.2. While diabetes prevalence was not related to socio-economic position in this study, the prevalence of diabetic eye disease, was higher among men and women residing in more deprived areas. Since good control of diabetes reduces the development of complications like diabetic eye disease differential experience of medical care for diabetes across socio-economic groups could contribute to the generation of this important inequity.

Unfortunately, most studies, in particularly randomised controlled trials, do not explicitly address the issue of whether medical interventions are of equal benefit regardless of socio-economic status. In addition, participants in trials are often unrepresentative of the general population. A recent re-analysis of the Multiple Risk Factor Intervention Trial clearly indicated an under-representation of poorer groups. However, despite the selection biases, limited evidence suggests that improvements in diastolic blood pressure, smoking cessation, and LDL-cholesterol, seen under trial conditions, are very similar for both well-educated and less-educated subjects; education being used as a marker of socio-economic status (Cutler & Grandits, 1995). The Hypertension Detection and Follow-up Program provides more compelling evidence that medical care can help address socio-economic differences in mortality by the appropriate management of hypertension (Hypertension Detection and Follow-up Program Cooperative Group, 1987). Amongst the group who received conventional medical care (referred care) there was a two-fold mortality gradient, based on whether the subject did, or did not receive high school education. In contrast, the special (stepped care) group showed almost non-existent gradients amongst both black and white subjects (see Figure 6.6). Similarly, the Systolic Hypertension in the Elderly Programme (SHEP) anti-hypertension trial also found similar reductions in cardiovascular mortality for different educational-level groups, with the less-educated group showing, if anything, larger benefits (Cutler & Grandits, 1995).

These data provide evidence on the efficacy of treatments but do not reflect the reality of day-to-day health care provision. Observational data consistently indicate that socio-demographic factors such as socio-economic position (Ben-Shlomo & Chaturvedi 1995), gender (Petticrew et al., 1993), ethnicity (Shaukat et al., 1993), and other factors such as smoking status (Morris et al., 1996), have an influence on the likelihood of receiving health interventions. This has been best documented in the US, where the two-tier health care system ensures a large vulnerable segment of the population who may not be able to afford major health care expenditure (Hayward et al., 1988). In England, it is assumed that a free health care system will not deter poorer

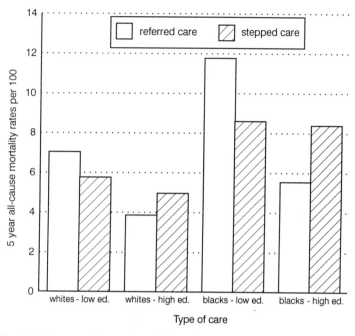

Fig. 6.6 Five-year all-cause mortality by educational level, race and intervention in the HDFP trial. (Adapted from Hypertension Detection and Follow-up Program Co-operative Group 1987.)

individuals from treatment. However, inequities appear to exist both for receiving surgery for heart disease (Ben-Shlomo & Chaturvedi, 1995) and other common surgical conditions (Chaturvedi & Ben-Shlomo, 1995). Men living in more affluent areas were more likely to receive coronary revascularisation surgery (see Fig. 6.7), despite having less need as measured by mortality rates (Ben-Shlomo & Chaturvedi, 1995). A more recent study has confirmed these findings with better data, indicating that people living in the most deprived wards had only about half the number of revascularisations per head of population with angina (Payne & Saul, 1997). In affluent wards, individuals with symptoms had almost three times the rate of coronary angiograms than those in poorer wards. Similarly, Asian patients with heart disease appear to wait almost twice as long from symptom onset to being seen by a cardiologist (Shaukat et al., 1993) as well as being less likely to receive thrombolytic therapy (Shaukat et al., 1997). Women are generally less likely to receive surgical intervention for heart

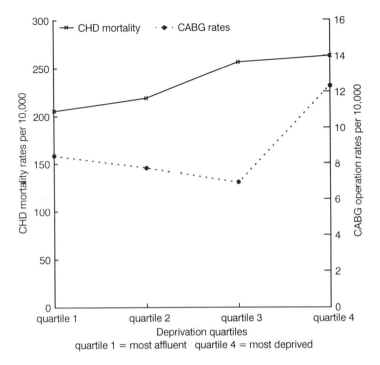

Fig. 6.7   Male mortality rates for coronary heart disease and coronary artery by-pass graft operation rates by deprivation quartiles. (Adapted from Ben-Shlomo & Chaturvedi 1995.)

disease (Steingart *et al.*, 1991). This is partially explained by the fact that they are more likely to have non-cardiac chest pain or less severe disease (Harris & Weissfeld 1991; Shaw *et al.*, 1994). However, amongst men and women with a past history of myocardial infarction, women still appear to be less likely to receive surgical intervention compared to men (Steingart *et al.*, 1991; Dong *et al.*, 1996), despite the fact that natural history studies suggest they have the same or worse prognosis as men (Weaver *et al.*, 1996).

Differences in access are not inevitable and have not always been found. In Northern Ireland, for example, no differences were noted in access to coronary revascularisation surgery by area deprivation (Kee *et al.*, 1993). A recent report from Finland, similarly failed to find differences in the survival of diabetics by socio-economic status (Koskinen, Martelin & Valkonen, 1996). Equitable health services has been an important goal in Finnish health policy for decades.

This suggests that health care purchasers must not only explicitly contract for equitable service provision but also take an active role in monitoring this both through routine health services activity data and clinical audit (Majeed *et al.*, 1994). One obvious and simple way of reducing potential inequities of service delivery is by the use of explicit guidelines. Whilst it is not always easy to get clinicians to apply guidelines, such a method, as in the stepped care approach used by the HDFP trial, may prevent demographic factors influencing the provision of health care, particularly if this is audited.

CONCLUSIONS

Inequalities in health in the UK are substantial and of increasing magnitude. The main way to address such health differentials is clearly through broader social and political changes leading to a more equitable society. Public health practitioners are failing in achieving their major objective — an improvement in population health status — if they do not become advocates for such changes.

REFERENCES

Albanes D, Jones D Y, Schatzkin A, Micozzi M S, Taylor P R 1988 Adult stature and risk of cancer. Cancer Research 48: 1658–62
Alter R, Riley J 1989 Frailty, sickness and death: Models of morbidity and mortality in historical populations. Population Studies 43: 25–46
Arblaster L, Lambert M, Entwistle V, Forster M, Fullerton D, Sheldon T, Watt I 1996. A systematic review of the effectiveness of health service interventions aimed at reducing inequalities in health. J Health Serv Res Policy 1: 93–103
Ashton J 1992 Healthy Cities. Open University Press, Milton Keynes
Barker D J P 1995 Early nutrition and coronary heart disease. In Nutrition in Child Health, ed. D P Davies, Royal College of Physicians of London, London
Bartley M, Power C, Blane D, Davey Smith G, Shipley M J 1994 Birthweight and later socio-economic disadvantage: evidence from the 1958 British cohort study. British Medical Journal 309: 1475–8
Ben-Shlomo Y, Chaturvedi N 1995 Assessing equity in access to health care provision in the UK: does where you live affect your chances of getting a coronary artery bypass graft? Journal of Epidemiology and Community Health 49: 200–4
Ben-Shlomo Y, and Davey Smith G 1991 Deprivation in infancy or in adult life: which is more important for mortality risk? Lancet 337: 530–4
Bentham G, Eimermann J, Haynes R, Lovett A, Brainaird J 1995 Limiting long term illness and its association with mortality and indicators of social deprivation. Journal of Epidemiology and Community Health 49 (Suppl. 2): S57-64
Blane D, Bartley M, Davey Smith G 1997 in press Disease aetiology and socio-economic mortality differentials. European Journal of Public Health
Blane D, Davey Smith G, Bartley M 1993 Social selection: what does it contribute to social class differences in health? Social Health Illness, 15: 1–15
Bosma H, Marmot M G, Hemingway H, Nicholson A C, Brunner E, Stansfeld S 1997 Low job control and risk of coronary heart disease. Whitehall II (prospective cohort) study, British Medical Journal 314: 558–65

Braverman H 1974 Labour and monopoly capital. Monthly Review Press, New York
Brunner E J, Marmot M G, White I R, O'Brien J R, Etherington M D, Slavin B M, Kearney E M, Davey Smith G 1993 Gender and employment grade differences in blood cholesterol, apolipoproteins and haemostatic factors in the Whitehall II study. Atherosclerosis 102: 195–207
Bunker J P, Frazier H S, Mosteller F 1995 The role of medical care in determining health: creating an inventory of benefits. In Society and Health ed. B C Amick, S Levine, A R Tarlov, D C Walsh OUP, New York
Cameron D, Jones I G 1985 An epidemiological and sociological analysis of the use of alcohol, tobacco, and other drugs of solace. Community Medicine 7: 18–29
Carroll D, Davey Smith G, Bennett P 1996 Some observations on health and socio-economic status. Journal of Health Psychology, 1: 23–39
Carstairs V, Morris R 1991 Deprivation and Health in Scotland. Aberdeen University Press, Aberdeen
Centerwell B S 1984 Race, socioeconomic status, and domestic homicide, Atlanta, 1971-72. American Journal of Public Health, 74: 813–15
Chaturvedi N, Ben-Shlomo Y 1995 From the surgery to the surgeon: does deprivation influence consultation and operation rates. British Journal of General Practice, 45: 127–31
Child Poverty Action Group 1996 Poverty: The facts. CPAG, London
Congdon P 1996 The epidemiology of suicide in London. Journal of the Royal Statistical Society 159: 515–33
Cutler J A, Grandits G 1995 What have we learned about socioeconomic status and cardiovascular disease from large trials? In Report of the conference on socioeconomic status and cardiovascular health and disease: November 6–7, 1995. ed. J Stamler, H P Hazuda Bethesda, Maryland: National Institutes of Health
Davey Smith G, Bartley M, Blane D 1990a The Black report on socioeconomic inequalities in health 10 years on. British Medical Journal 301: 373–7
Davey Smith G, Carroll D, Rankin S, Rowan D 1992 Socioeconomic differentials in mortality: evidence from Glasgow graveyards. British Medical Journal 305: 1554–7
Davey Smith G, Bartley M, Blane D 1994a Explanations for socio-economic differentials in mortality: evidence from Britain and elsewhere. European Journal of Public Health 4: 131–44
Davey Smith G, Hart C, Hole D, Gillis C, Watt G, Hawthorne V 1994b Education and occupational social class: which is the more important indicator of mortality risk? (Abstract). Journal of Epidemiology and Community Health 48: 500
Davey Smith G, Kuh D 1996 Does early nutrition affect later health: views from the 1930s and 1980s. In The History of Nutrition in Britain in the Twentieth Century: Science, Scientists and Politics. ed D Smith, Routledge
Davey Smith G, Morris J 1994 Increasing inequalities in the health of the nation (editorial). British Medical Journal 309: 1453–4
Davey Smith G, Shipley M J, Rose G 1990b The magnitude and causes of socio-economic differentials in mortality: further evidence from the Whitehall study. Journal of Epidemiology and Community Health 44: 260–5
Davey Smith G, Shipley M J 1991 Confounding of occupation and smoking: its magnitude and consequences. Social Science Medicine 32: 1297–300
Davey Smith G, Brunner E 1997 Socio-economic differentials in health: the role of nutrition. Proceedings of the Nutrition Society 56: 75–90
Davey Smith G, Hart C, Blane D, Gillis C, Hawthorne V 1997 Lifetime socioeconomic position and mortality: prospective observational study. British Medical Journal 314: 547–52
Department of Health 1995 Variations in Health: What can the Department of Health and the NHS do? Department of Health, London
Department of Health 1996 Low Income, Food, Nutrition and Health: strategies for improvement. Department of Health, London
Diez-Roux A V, Nieto F J, Tyroler H A, Crum L D, Szklo M 1995 Social inequali-

98 PROGRESS IN PUBLIC HEALTH

ties and atherosclerosis. The atherosclerosis risk in communities study. *American Journal of Epidemiology* 141: 960–72

Dong W, Colhoun H, Ben-Shlomo Y, Chaturvedi N 1996 Cardiac surgery in England — do men and women have equal access? (abstract) Journal of Epidemiology and Community Health 50: 590–1

Dowler E 1996 Women and food in poor families: focus for concern? In Focus on Women: Nutrition and health. ed J Bultriss, K Hyman London: National Dairy Council, London

Drever F, Whitehead M, Roden M 1996 Current patterns and trends in male mortality by social class (based on occupation) population trends 86: 15–20

Eachus J, Williams M, Chan P, Davey Smith G, Grainge M, Donovan J, Frankel S 1996 Deprivation and cause-specific morbidity: evidence from the Somerset and Avon Survey of Health. British Medical Journal 312: 287–92

Egolf B, Lasker J, Wolf S, Potvin L 1992 The Roseto effect: a 50-year comparison of mortality rates. American Journal of Public Health 82: 1089–92

Elo I T, Preston S H 1996 Educational differentials in mortality: United States, 1979–85. Social Science Medicine, 42: 47–57.

Elstad J I 1996 How large are the differences really? Self-reported long-standing illness among working class and middle class men. Sociology of Health and Illness 18: 475–98

Engels F 1845, 1987 The condition of the working class in England. Penguin, Harmondsworth

Foster P 1996 Inequalities in health: what health systems can and cannot do. Journal of Health Services Research and Policy, 1: 179–82

Frankel S, Elwood P, Sweetnam P, Yarnell J, Davey Smith G 1996 Birthweight, body-mass index in middle age, and incident coronary heart disease. Lancet 348: 1478–80

Glynn A and Miliband D 1994 Paying for Inequality: The economic cost of social justice. Rivers Oram Press, London

Goldman L, Cook E F 1984 The decline in ischemic heart disease mortality rates. An analysis of the comparative effects of medical interventions and changes in lifestyle. Annals of Internal Medicine, 101: 825–36.

Graham H 1988 Women and smoking in the UK *Health Promotion* 3: 371–82

Gunnell D, Davey Smith G, Frankel S, Nanchahal K, Braddon F E M, Pemberton J, Peters T J 1996 Childhood leg length and adult mortality — follow up of the Carnegie (Boyd Orr) Survey of diet and growth in pre-war Britain. Journal of Epidemiology and Community Health 50: 580–1

Haan M, Kaplan G A, Camacho T 1987 Poverty and health: prospective evidence from the Alameda County study. American Journal of Epidemiology, 125: 989–98

Harding S. (1995). Social class differences in mortality of men: recent evidence from the OPCS Longitudinal Study. Population Trends 80: 31–7

Harris R B, Weissfeld L A 1991 Gender differences in the reliability of reporting symptoms of angina pectoris. Journal of Clinical Epidemiology 44: 1071–8

Hart C, Ecob R & Davey Smith G 1997 People, places and coronary heart disease risk factors: a multilevel analysis of the Scottish heart health study archive. Social Science Medicine 45; 893–902

Hayward R A, Shapiro M F, Freeman H E, Corey C R 1988 Inequities in health services among insured Americans. New England Journal of Medicine 318; 1507–12

Hertzman C 1996 What's been said and what's been hid: population health, global consumption and the role of national health data systems. In Health and Social Organization: towards a health policy for the 21st century. Routledge, London eds D Blane, E Brunner, R Wilkinson

Hertzman C, Wiens M 1996 Child development and long term outcomes: a population health perspective and summary of successful interventions. *Social Science Medicine* 43: 1083-95

Holme I, Helgeland A, Hjermann I, Leren P, Lund-Larsen P G 1980. Four-year mortality by some socio-economic indicators: the Oslo study. Journal of Epidemiology and Community Health 34: 48–52

Hypertension Detection and Follow-up Program Cooperative Group 1987 Education level and 5-year all-cause mortality in the HDFP. Hypertension 9: 641–6

Jones H B 1956 A special consideration of the ageing process, disease and life-expectancy. Advances in Biology and Medical Physics 4: 281–337

Jones K, Duncan C 1995 Individuals and their ecologies: analysing the geography of chronic illness within a multilevel modelling framework. *Health and Place*, 1: 27–40

Kee F, Gaffney B, Currie S, O'Reilly D 1993 Access to coronary catheterisation: fair shares for all? British Medical Journal 307: 1305–7

Koskinen S 1994 Origins of regional differences in mortality from ischaemic heart disease in Finland. National Research and Development Centre for Welfare and Health Search Report 41. NAWH, Helsinki

Koskinen, S V P, Martelin T P, Valkonen T 1996 Socioeconomic differences in mortality among diabetic people in Finland: five year follow up. British Medical Journal 313: 975–8

Kuh D, Davey Smith, G 1993 When is mortality risk determined? Historical insights into a current debate. Social History of Medicine 6: 101–23

Leitch I. 1951 Growth and Health. British Journal of Nutrition 5: 142–151.

Lobstein T. 1995. The increasing cost of a healthy diet. Food Mag., 31: 17

Lynch J W, Kaplan GA, Cohen RD, Tuomilehto J, Salonen JT 1996 Do known risk factors explain the relation between socioeconomic status, risk of all-cause mortality, cardiovascular mortality and acute myocardial infarction? American Journal of Epidemiology 144: 934-42

Mackenbach J P, Bouvier-Colle M H, Jougla E 1990 'Avoidable' mortality and health services: a review of aggregate data studies. Journal of Epidemiology and Community Health 44: 106–11

Mackenbach J P, Looman C W N, van der Meer J B W 1996 Differences in the mis-reporting of chronic conditions, by level of education: effect on inequalities in prevalence rates American Journal of Public Health 86: 706–11

Majeed F A, Chaturvedi N, Reading R, Ben-Shlomo Y 1994 Equity in the NHS: Monitoring and promoting equity in primary and secondary care. British Medical Journal 308: 1426–9

Mare R D 1990 Socioeconomic careers and differential mortality among older men in the United Stages. In Measurement and Analysis of Mortality: New Approaches. ed. J Vallin, S D'Douza, A Palloni Clarendon Press, Oxford, England pp.362–87

Marmot M G, Davey Smith G, Stansfeld S, Patel C, North F, Head J, White I, Brunner E, Feeney A 1991 Inequalities in health twenty years on: the Whitehall II study of British Civil Servants. Lancet 337: 1387–94

Marmot M, Bobak M, Davey Smith G, 1995 Explanations for social inequalities in health. In Society and Health. ed BC Amick, S Levine, A Tarlov, DC Walsh Oxford University Press.

McKeown T, Record R G, Turner R D 1975 An interpretation of the decline of mortality in England and Wales during the twentieth century. Population Studies 29: 391–421

Morris R W, McCallum A K, Walker M, Whincup P H, Ebrahim S, Shaper A G 1996 Cigarette smoking in British men and selection for coronary artery bypass surgery. Heart 75: 557–62

Pamuk E R 1985 Social class inequality and mortality from 1921–1971 in England and Wales. Population Studies 39: 17–31

Patrick D, Wickizer T M 1995 Community and Health. In Society and Health. ed B C Amick, S Levine, A R Tarlov, D C Walsh, Oxford University Press, New York

Payne N Saul C 1997 Variations in use of cardiology services in a health authority: comparison of coronary artery revascularisation rates with prevalence of angina and coronary mortality. British Medical Journal 314: 257–61

Petticrew M, McKee M, Jones J 1993 Coronary artery surgery: are women discriminated against? British Medical Journal 306: 1164–6

Phillimore P, Beattie A, Townsend P 1994 Widening inequality of health in Northern England, 1981–91. British Medical Journal 308: 1125–8

Putnam R D, Leonardi R, Nanetti R Y 1993 Making democracy work: civic traditions in modern Italy. Princeton University Press, Princeton, N J

Rowett Research Institute 1955 Family Diet and Health in Pre-war Britain. Carnegie United Kingdom Trust, Dunfermline

Salhi M, Caselli G, Duchêne J, Egidi V, Santini A, Thiltgés E, Wunsch G 1995 Assessing mortality differentials using life histories: a method and applications. In ed A Lopez, G Caselli, T Valkonen. Adult Mortality in Developed Countries: From description to explanation. Oxford: Clarendon Press

Shaukat N, de Bono D P, Cruickshank J K 1993 Clinical features, risk factors, and referral delay in British patients of Indian and European origin with angina matched for age and extent of coronary atheroma. British Medical Journal 307: 717–18

Shaukat N, Lear J, Lowy A, Fletcher S, de Bono D P, Woods K L 1997 First myocardial infarction in patients of Indian subcontinent and European origin: comparison of risk factors, management, and long term outcome. British Medical Journal 314: 639–42

Shaw L J, Miller D D, Romeis J C, Kargl D, Younis L T, Chaitman B R 1994 Gender differences in the noninvasive evaluation and management of patients with suspected coronary artery disease. Annals of Internal Medicine 1994;120: 559–66

Shouls S, Congdon P, Curtis S 1996 Modelling inequality in reported long term illness in the UK: combining individual and area characteristics. Journal of Epidemiology and Community Health 50: 366–76

Sloggett A, Joshi H 1994 Higher mortality in deprived areas: community or personal disadvantage. British Medical Journal 309: 1470–74

Sooman, A, Macintyre S 1995 Health and perceptions of the local environment in socially contrasting neighbourhoods in Glasgow. Health and Place, 1: 15–26

Sooman A, Macintyre S, Anderson A 1993 Scotland's health: A more difficult challenge for some? Health Bulletin 51: 276–284

Steingart R M, Packer M, Hamm P et al. 1991 Sex differences in the management of coronary artery disease. New England Journal of Medicine 325: 226–30

Tannenbaum A 1947 Effects of varying caloric intake upon tumor incidence and tumor growth. Annals of the NY Academy of Science 49: 5–18

Travers K D (1996). The social organisation of nutritional inequalities. Social Science Medicine 43: 543-53

Tyroler H A, Wing S, Knowles M G 1993 Increasing inequality in coronary heart disease mortality in relation to educational achievement profiles of places of residence, United States, 1962 to 1987. Annals of Epidemiology 3 (suppl): S51–4

Vague J 1956 The degree of masculine differentiation of obesities: a factor determining predisposition to diabetes, atherosclerosis, gout, and uric calculous disease. American Journal of Clinical Nutrition 4: 20–34

Valkonen T 1987 Male mortality from ischaemic heart disease in Finland, relation to region of birth and region of residence. European Journal of Population 3: 61–83

Weaver W D, White H D, Wilcox R G, et al. 1996 Comparisons of characteristics and outcomes among women and men with acute myocardial infarction treated with thrombolytic therapy. Journal of the American Medical Association 275: 777–82

Whitehead M 1992 The health divide. In Inequalities in Health. ed P Townsend, N Davidson, M Whitehead. Penguin books, Harmondsworth

7. Recent Developments in the Geographical Analysis of Small Area Health and Environmental Data

Paul Elliott and David Briggs

INTRODUCTION

Traditionally, geographical analyses have been used to describe broad-scale differences in disease risk across large geographical areas, for example, the well-known regional differences in mortality and the incidence of coronary heart disease in Great Britain (higher rates in the north of England, and in Scotland, compared with the South-East and South-West). More recently, attention has focused on local (small area) variations in disease risk. The reasons for this shift in geographical scale can be summarised as follows:

- public concern about environmental causes of disease, especially environmental pollution, and heightened awareness about possible disease 'clusters';
- requirement of Directors of Public Health to report on the disease experience of their populations, typically (though not exclusively) including small area disease mapping to highlight areas at apparently increased risk;
- availability of routine health statistics with high resolution geographical coding, e.g., the postcode of residence in the UK;
- availability of small area statistics from census giving population counts and other socio-demographic data at small area scale (enumeration district in the UK);
- massive improvements in computing power and database technology allowing rapid retrieval and analysis of large volumes of data at reasonable cost;
- development of geographical information system (GIS) techniques for the handling, interrogation and display of geo-

graphical data, and the widespread availability of 'user friend-ly' GIS software.

In this chapter, we discuss sources of routine data in the UK available for small area analyses — not only health and population data, but also possible 'explanatory' variables, i.e. other socio-demographic and environmental data. We then review the application of geographical methods, and in particular GIS, to the health field, and outline the strengths but also the weaknesses of the approach. Finally, we briefly examine three common applications of small area geographical methods: cluster investigation, disease mapping, and small area geographic correlation studies of environment and health. Advances in the relevant statistical methodology are reviewed elsewhere (Alexander & Boyle, 1996; Alexander & Cuzick 1992; Clayton & Bernardinelli, 1992; Elliott *et al.*, 1995; Olsen *et al.*, 1996).

Definition of Small Area

First, however, it seems appropriate to define the term 'small area'. In fact, no satisfactory definition exists. In the context of environmental health 'small area' has sometimes been used to describe an analysis carried out at sub-national or perhaps sub-regional level, i.e. at a geographical scale below that of the standard (published) reporting of disease rates. This definition takes no account of population size, which may differ substantially between areas, or disease frequency, and is therefore of limited use. Putative disease 'clusters', for example, are unlikely to respect administrative boundaries for which population data or health statistics are reported. Any disease excess may occur on a much finer geographical scale or cross arbitrary geographical boundaries — the leukaemia 'cluster' at Seascale near the Sellafield nuclear plant is a case in point. Under such circumstances, a purely local excess is unlikely to be detected in the routine statistics.

A more useful definition would take into account the number of cases observed, which itself would depend on population size, disease frequency and time-period of analysis. As a rough guide, Cuzick and Elliott (1992) suggested that any geographical area containing fewer than about 20 cases of disease could be considered a small area. As many cancers have annual incidence rates of around 5 per 100,000, over a five-year period, a small area might comprise a population of around 100,000 or less. For rare diseases or small populations in rural areas, the population size might be much less, but usually populations of at least 10,000 or so are required to form an aggregation of minimal size (Cuzick & Elliott, 1992). Of course, populations of individual areas could be much smaller if the disease distribution across many such areas is of primary interest, for example, in small-area disease mapping (see p.116).

DATA

In this section, we briefly review some of the data that have been used in small area geographical studies of health and the environment. As with all types of epidemiological enquiry, geographical studies are subject to a number of problems related to the availability, quality and applicability of the data. A detailed appreciation of the nature and quality of the various data sources (health, population, environment) is necessary for proper understanding and interpretation of geographical analyses. For example, apparent geographical variations in disease could reflect differences between populations in case definition, completeness of ascertainment, diagnostic accuracy, coding or (for mortality) survival rates; and population estimates (necessary for the calculation of disease rates) may be distorted by incomplete enumeration of the population (e.g. at census) or by recent migration.

Health Data

In Europe, notably the UK and the Scandinavian countries, a number of routine health datasets are available that include a high resolution geographical code. This is usually place of residence, but in some cases there is the possibility of linking to other relevant locations, such as place of birth. In the Scandinavian countries, this is achieved by using the unique person number to identify each individual. In the UK, as noted earlier, the postcode of residence is used. There are currently around 2 million postcodes in the UK. Each postcode relates to only 14 households on average, and its 'centroid' can be located as a point on a map to 100 m accuracy. (Recent work by the Ordnance Survey called Address Point can locate each residential address to 1 m accuracy, although currently this is not routinely available for epidemiological enquiries as the costs are prohibitive.)

Sources of routinely postcoded data nationally in Great Britain are summarised in Table 7.1, together with comments on their utility for small area analyses. While all-cause mortality data are essentially complete, there may be considerable variability in the accuracy of cause-specific mortality. In contrast with deaths (and births) there is no statutory notification of cancer incidence, so that

Table 7.1 Examples of routinely postcoded health and vital statistics data in Great Britain

Data	Year (from)	Source (national*)	Comment
Mortality	1981 (E&W) 1974 (Scotland)	ONS GRO(S)	Complete, but diagnostic accuracy and coding of underlying cause of death may vary.
Cancer incidence	1974 (E&W) 1975 (Scotland)	ONS ISD	Various degrees of under-ascertainment and duplication, both between registries and at sub-regional level. The quality of the national register has improved in recent years.
Congenital malformations	1983 (E&W) 1988 (Scotland)†	ONS ISD	Major problem of under-ascertainment in national register. Some specialised local registries have much higher levels of ascertainment. A high quality database is being produced in Scotland.
Hospital Episode Statistics (England) and Scottish Morbidity Record	1991 (England) 1981 (Scotland)	DoH ISD	Huge database (c. 10 million records/year in England). Episode, not person based in England. Diagnostic accuracy, coding, etc. varies between hospitals. Linked individual database available in Scotland.
Births	1981 (E&W) 1974 (Scotland)	ONS GRO(S)	Complete. Provides postcoded denominator for early childhood events.
Stillbirths	1981 (E&W) 1974 (Scotland)	ONS GRO(S)	Data on stillbirths complete, but data on early and late abortions not routinely available.

* Some of these data may be available from local sources, e.g. district health authorities, regional offices and regional cancer registries, or hospital trusts, i.e. hospital episode statistics.
† Available from mid-1997.
E&W England and Wales.
ONS Office for National Statistics.
GRO(S) General Register Office, Scotland.
ISD Information and Statistics Division of the National Health Service in Scotland.
DoH Department of Health (England).

under-ascertainment is a potential source of error with those data. In addition, duplicate entries occur, which may be a particular problem for small area analyses since even one or two duplicates of a rare cancer could result in an apparent disease 'cluster' in a particular area. Thus any small area investigation of cancer statistics should usually include some data validation. A specialised national cancer registry for children, with high levels of clinical input and quality control, holds postcoded national data from the 1960s (maintained by the Childhood Cancer Research Group in Oxford).

Hospital episode data are a newly available resource for small area analysis, although there are considerable constraints to their routine use. The problems include diagnostic completeness and accuracy, variation in quality and completeness of the coding, and variable interpretation of the coding rules themselves. In Scotland, a validated database has linked data for individuals dating from 1981. In England, the data are episode rather than person based, although approximate linkages can be achieved using date of birth, sex and postcode. Despite the problems, the hospital data offer exciting new possibilities for carrying out small area analyses of contemporary data relating to current potential exposures, for example, acute admissions for asthma in relation to traffic-related air pollution (Wilkinson *et al.*, 1997a). This is in contrast to analyses of mortality or cancer incidence, which, for the most part, relate to putative exposures encountered many years previously, due to the long latency between exposure and outcome.

Congenital malformation data held on the national registry (maintained for England and Wales by the Office for National Statistics) are currently of limited value for small area analyses because of the high levels of under-ascertainment. Thus evidence of geographical variability could point to 'troughs' of under-ascertainment rather than 'peaks' of excess incidence. However it is to be hoped that recent interest in improving the quality of the national data will result in a usable small-area database for at least some conditions, e.g. Down syndrome. In Scotland, a high quality database for congenital anomalies, from 1988, should be available towards the latter part of 1997. In addition, high quality specialised malformation registers already exist in some areas, and these are a valuable potential resource for small area study.

National data shown in Table 7.1 are held by the UK Small Area Health Statistics Unit (SAHSU). This was established following a government enquiry into the alleged cluster of leukaemia in children and young people near Sellafield (Black, 1984). Its terms of reference include to: respond rapidly to reports of disease excess ('clusters') near sources of environmental pollution; carry out studies of health statistics more generally around sources of pollution; carry out descriptive geographical studies at small-area level; and develop the methodology. Plans are advanced to set up a rapid response facility which could offer District Health Authorities basic geographical analyses (e.g. observed/expected ratios) for defined small areas or around specified points. Recent epidemiological enquiries carried out by SAHSU include an investigation of cancer incidence and mortality near a pesticide factory, following media reports of excess cancers in the vicinity (Wilkinson *et al.*, 1997b), and national studies of cancer incidence near municipal solid waste incinerators (Elliott *et al*.,1996) and near radio and television transmitters (Dolk *et al.*, 1997 a,b).

Population data

In the UK, population data for small areas (enumeration districts) are available from national census. A typical enumeration district gives population counts (by sex, in five-year age groups) and socio-economic data for about 400 people and enables appropriate standardisation to be carried out, i.e. the calculation of a standardised mortality (or morbidity) ratio (SMR) by small area. However, no reliable small-area population estimates are published for the intercensal years. In the future, it is to be expected that general practice population data for Health Authority and Board area may become an important subsidiary source of population data.

In the absence of such data on annual counts, many studies currently rely on constructing a 'data window' around each census, and apply census-year population counts over several different years. Although errors are likely to be small when populations are aggregated up to larger areas, this is not the case for small-area analyses where large errors in population estimation can occur (Diamond, 1992), for example, in areas of rapid development, or where there was substantial under-enumeration at census (e.g. for young single men in inner city areas). Again, even if the population size remains stable over time, no allowance is made for in- and out-migration, which can be extensive especially in inner city areas. This will effectively reduce the size of the population at risk, and hence could bias downward estimates of risk.

In England and Wales (though not in Scotland), only approximate links exist between postcodes (i.e. event data) and enumeration districts (population data), introducing an extra source of error into the calculation of the SMR. In a small proportion of cases, postcodes themselves may be wrong or inaccurately located. The sum total of these sources of error in the population data is to add a further degree of uncertainty into estimates of disease risk. However, any bias is unlikely to be more than, say, +/- 5%, which is generally within acceptable limits for small area studies of this kind.

Environmental Data

Problems of data availability are generally more severe when exposure data are considered. Relevant measures are often lacking, both at the level of individuals and for ecological analyses. Individual exposure sampling and biological monitoring are both costly and invasive, even where reliable and valid measures to estimate exposure are available. Environmental monitoring is also expensive and is likely to give only a partial picture of true exposure over an area, especially if it is exposure integrated over many years that is of most interest.

Responsibility for environmental monitoring in the UK resides with a wide range of agencies, including government bodies, local authorities and public utilities. Arrangements for monitoring vary between England and Wales, Scotland and Northern Ireland, and the extent and structure of monitoring networks tend to change constantly, in response to new legislative requirements, technological innovations, and the changing condition of the environment. For these reasons, any summary of the status of environmental data tends to be incomplete and soon out of date.

Table 7.2 lists some of the main national data sources of potential interest for small-area health applications. Local authorities also collect a considerable variety of environmental data, either under their statutory obligations, or for local management purposes. These have not been included here, however, because details vary from one authority to another, and in any case there is no readily available inventory of data collected.

Use of these data for small area health applications faces a number of difficulties. Whilst most national data are subject to rigorous quality controls, and are likely to be broadly consistent, problems of equipment failure, changes in site location and methodology, and the different purposes and designs of different monitoring networks mean that environmental data must be used and interpreted with caution. Data on atmospheric emissions present particular problems as emission factors are often adjusted in the light of new information

Table 7.2 Examples of national, routine environmental data

Medium	Pollutants/indicator	Source	Description
Atmospheric emissions	Annual emissions of: Black smoke Sulphur dioxide Nitrogen oxides Non-methane VOCs CO CO_2 Methane	AEA Technology	Emission estimates for mid–late 1980s for 10 km × 10 km grid across UK (1km × 1km grid for London); from major point, line and diffuse sources; updated irregularly
Air quality	Sulphur dioxide concentration	AEA Technology	23 automatic sites; 308 active sampler sites (38 rural)
	Black smoke concentration	DoE	270 active sampler sites
	Fine particulate concentration		14 automatic sites
	Nitrogen dioxide concentration		26 automatic sites, c. 1200 diffusion tube sites
	Lead concentration		13 active sampler sites
	Ozone concentration		31 automatic sites (14 rural 17 urban)
	Carbon monoxide concentration		21 automatic sites
Stream water quality	Biological water classification	Environment Agency	All stream segments classified on A (good) to D (poor) scale, based on the macroinvertebrate species present in the streams
	General water quality classification		All major streams classified on A (good) – F (bad) scale, based on measurements of BOD, dissolved oxygen and ammonia concentration
Surface water pollution incidents	Number of pollution incidents		Number of incidents by source, severity and outcome (by site)
Groundwater quality	Nitrates and pesticide concentrations		National network in process of development
Bathing water quality	Number and percentage of bathing waters complying with coliform standard during the bathing season		Status of bathing waters for c. 457 sites in UK
Drinking water quality	Percentage of determinations exceeding PCV	Water companies	Statistical results of water testing in areas with up to 50,000 inhabitants (c. 2.8 million determinations for c. 18 major parameters in 1992)

Table 7.2 *continued*

Medium	Pollutants/ indicator	Source	Description
Radon	Mean annual and peak indoor concentration; number and percentage of houses above the Radon Action Level (200 Bq/m³)	National Radiological Protection Board	Stratified survey of houses in UK (*c.* 270,000 dwellings by 1996)
Radioactivity	Average gamma radiation dose	DoE	Hourly measurements at 46 sites (up to 1992); increased to 92 sites in 1993

Source: DoE, Department of Environment (1996); Bower & Vallence-Plews (1995).
AEA, Atomic Energy Authority.
BOD, Biological Oxygen Demand.
PCV, Prescribed Concentration Value.
VOC, Volatile Organic Compounds.

on emission rates and combustion performance: between 1983 and 1993, national emission factors for nitrogen dioxide (NO_2), for example, were adjusted on no fewer than ten occasions, resulting in an almost 50% increase in estimated emission rates (Briggs 1995). Air quality monitoring networks have also been established for different purposes (e.g. to meet statutory requirements, to guide policy, for public information, or for research purposes). These may imply different siting criteria and analytical techniques, so that data from different networks are not necessarily comparable. Analysis of the 270 sites currently monitoring atmospheric black smoke and SO_2 shows that fewer than 120 achieved an 80% data capture rate in at least 80% of years over the period 1981 and 1995.

As another example, the national stream water quality classification was fundamentally changed in the early 1990s, making direct comparisons with earlier years difficult. The length of streams surveyed has also changed over the years, primarily through the inclusion of more smaller and less polluted stream reaches; this has tended to exaggerate the apparent improvements in stream water quality.

Notwithstanding these limitations, it is evident that the range and quality of environmental information in the UK has improved considerably over recent years. To a large extent, this is due to improvements in technologies for ground-based monitoring. In the case of air pollution, one example of this has been the rapid expansion of automatic monitoring networks in the UK, covering SO_2, NO_x and ozone. By 1992, these comprised 34 sites, including six sites as part of an enhanced urban network (EUN), located in some of the worst affected city centres. By 1997, the EUN will expand to 24 sites, and ultimately it is planned to establish a network of 80 automatic sites in urban areas in the UK. At the same time, another important development has been in the design of low-cost monitoring devices, such as diffusion tubes and badges. Devices capable of measuring ambient concentrations of nitrogen dioxide have been available for many years, but are now being extended to a range of other pollutants, including SO_2, CO, NH_3, formaldehyde and ozone (Williams, 1995). While they cannot command the accuracy of traditional fixed-site monitoring systems (precision of c. 6–12% is often quoted for SO_2, 10–20% for formaldehyde and c. 5–15% for NO_2 (Noy et al., 1990; van Reeuwijk et al., 1997)), none the less, they offer the considerable advantage of cheapness and ease of deployment. This means that they can be used for intensive survey campaigns, and can provide the spatial coverage and density which traditional monitoring devices cannot give, making them potentially of value for small-area applications. As an example, a major national campaign has been carried out in the UK, using diffusion tubes for NO_2 (Campbell et al., 1994). Continuously recording personal analysers are also becoming available for a range of pollutants, including NO_2, CO, ozone and SO_2, which offer considerable improvements over previous devices (Williams, 1995).

Similar advances are occurring in the monitoring of other environmental media. Until recently, for example, monitoring of stream water quality relied largely on manual sampling. This greatly restricted the frequency of sampling and meant that major pollution episodes could often be missed, and that identification and prosecution of the polluters was often difficult. Increasingly, however, these are being replaced or supplemented by continuous water samplers, which provide instantaneous analysis for a wide range of pollutants, and which are linked electronically, thereby allowing samplers to be triggered automatically in response to a pollution incident.

At the same time, important technological advances have been made in remote sensing. Satellite imagery represents a rich, although as yet under-used, source of data for health studies. Perhaps its greatest potential lies in mapping emission sources and activities (e.g. associated with agricultural activity, industry or transport) or health hazards related to land cover. Glass et al. (1995), for example, used satellite data to map areas of forest and other habitat types associated with the tick, Ixodes scapularis, as a basis for assessing risk of Lyme disease. Land cover data might similarly be useful for identifying exposures to pollen (e.g. from natural vegetation, agricultural grasses or oilseed rape), or to agricultural chemicals (e.g. pesticides). Equally, however, land cover data can also be used to help map the small-area distribution of population on the basis of the distribution and character of residential land (Langford *et al.*, 1991). The current generation of satellites provides greatly enhanced data on land cover for such applications — the SPOT satellites, for example, have a spatial resolution of c. 10 metres in panchromatic and c. 20 metres in colour, compared with resolutions of 40–50 metres from the previous Landsat imagery. In addition, new sensors are offering the capability for remote measurement of environmental pollution — for example, by the detection and tracking of marine oil pollution, smog episodes and soil pollution associated with landfill sites.

These developments in the availability and quality of environmental data imply greatly enhanced potential for correlating such exposures to health data, in so-called geographic correlation studies. Whilst intuitively attractive, such studies also have the potential to be seriously misleading if carried out naïvely, without due regard to the correlated structure of the data and the potential for confounding. This is discussed further below.

GEOGRAPHIC INFORMATION SYSTEMS

The range of health, population and environmental data outlined above takes many different forms. Data on both population and health outcome, for example, may relate to individual locations (points), such as the postcode centroid of place of residence, or to geographic areas (e.g. the census enumeration district or ward). Environmental data are often even more diverse. Data on air pollution, for instance, may be represented as point measurements (e.g. at fixed-site monitoring stations), as lines (e.g. roadways), as irregular polygons (e.g. modelled pollution plumes around major combustion sources) or as a regular grid (e.g. emission estimates for a 1 km grid across a city). The analysis of each of these different types of spatial data may require different methodologies. In many cases, also, there is a need to bring together, combine and convert between spatially discordant data sets. This need arises most acutely when environmental and health data are being integrated or compared, for these are rarely based on comparable spatial structures. Even in the case of supposedly coherent statistics, such as census data, similar difficulties may arise because of changes to the reporting units (e.g. enumeration districts) over time.

Environmental and health data are also often spatially discontinuous: they are based on sample designs which provide only a partial coverage of the entire area of interest. For many applications, such data need to be converted to continuous coverages. As noted previously, for example, surveys of air pollution levels within a city may be carried out using low-cost monitoring devices, such as diffusion tubes. In order to estimate population exposures, these point measurements need to be converted to a pollution map, which can then be overlaid on the population distribution. This requires the estimation of pollution levels at unsampled points, using some form of spatial interpolation.

Until recently, these and other types of spatial data manipulation posed serious computational difficulties. In recent years, however, the capability to handle large and complex spatial data sets has been fundamentally transformed by the development of GIS. Geographic information systems may be defined as systems for the manipulation and presentation of geo-referenced (i.e. spatial) data. As such, they are able to perform a range of functions, including:

- *data capture*: the acquisition of the data in digital form, e.g. by manual encoding, digitising or scanning;
- *data cleaning*: the checking, correction and editing of data to remove errors during data capture or transfer;
- *data integration*: a series of operations (e.g. generalisation, projection conversion, registration) which convert the data to a consistent geographical structure;
- *data storage*: holding the data in a geographically-referenced database in a form suitable for easy retrieval and analysis;
- *data search and retrieval*: the identification and recall of data on the basis of specific conditions defined by the user;
- *spatial analysis*: the geographical manipulation and transformation of the data (e.g. buffering, point-in-polygon analysis, interpolation, map overlay, network analysis);
- *statistical analysis*: the computation of descriptive statistics for either single or multiple geographical coverages;
- *visualisation*: the generation and display of maps or other output (graphs, tables, etc) either on screen or as hard copy.

These capabilities have made GIS a powerful tool in many different areas of application including health. Over the last 5–10 years, the use of GIS in health studies and health management has expanded greatly, and many health authorities in the UK have now adopted GIS, at least for the purpose of routine data presentation and analysis. A wide range of specialist research applications have also developed, notably for small-area health mapping, for the investigation of point patterns and clustering in health data, for the modelling and mapping of pollution, for exposure estimation, and to analyse relationships between environmental risk factors and health outcome (Briggs & Elliott, 1995).

One of the potentially most fruitful — yet also controversial — areas of application to health data has been in the detection of spatial patterns of disease by searching for spatial clustering within point data sets. An early example of this approach was provided by Openshaw et al. (1987, 1990), who developed a 'geographical analysis machine' (GAM) which systematically constructed buffer zones around a fixed lattice of points in the study area. If the number of observed cases exceeded a certain expected number, then a circle was drawn. Following repeated scanning with circles of different radius, the results were mapped, and locations which provided the focus for a large number of overlapping circles were identified as a disease 'cluster'. This approach has been heavily criticised, not least because of the problems of double counting and the lack of a theoretical basis for testing for 'true' excesses within complex spatial data sets.

Applications such as GAM illustrate well both the strengths and weaknesses of the GIS approach. On the one hand, GIS offers a powerful tool for the analysis and display of complex geographically organised data; on the other, the lack of a strong statistical foundation, coupled with visually appealing and often striking graphical display, can readily lead to over-interpretation, or, worse, misleading or false conclusions about underlying spatial relationships, e.g. between environmental factors and health.

An alternative approach, which allows for formal statistical testing, is provided by the use of a K-function. In health applications, this would comprise an analysis of the relative risk of disease based on the spatial distribution of pairs of points (i.e. cases and controls) at different locations. This has been used by Gattrell et al. (1991), within a procedure called Mikhail (Mission Impossible K-hat in ArcInfo at Lancaster), to estimate K functions in an investigation of spatial clustering in motor neurone disease. Gatrell and Rowlingson (1995) also illustrate the use of this method to investigate gastrointestinal infection in Lancaster.

Another common use of GIS has been in the mapping of pollution and exposure estimation. The spatial interpolation techniques available in GIS, for example, provide a powerful means for generating pollution maps on the basis of data from point measurement sites. One of the most widely adopted group of techniques in this context is kriging (Oliver & Webster, 1990; Wartenberg, 1993). These are based on regionalised variable theory, which state that the spatial variation in any variable can be expressed as:

$$Z(x) = m(x) + \epsilon'(x) + \epsilon''$$

where Z is a regionalised variable, x is the location, $m(x)$ is the structural component of variation (trend), $\epsilon'(x)$ is a stochastic, spatially dependent residual from $m(x)$, and ϵ'' is the residual, spatially independent component or noise. Kriging proceeds by first exploring the stochastic surface through the construction of a so-called semivariogram, then applying this to predict conditions at unsampled sites. In recent years, kriging techniques have gained a considerable following, and kriging routines are now included in a number of proprietary GIS, including ArcInfo. Kriging in its various forms has thus been used to map the distribution of radon gas (Vincent & Gatrell, 1991), ozone pollution (Lefohn et al., 1988; Liu et al., 1995), nitrogen dioxide (Campbell et al., 1994) and cyanide and cadmium pollution (Stein et al., 1995).

GIS also provides powerful tools for environmental and health planning and risk assessment. By combining data on the road network, population distribution, vehicle accidents and groundwater vulnerability, for example, Brainard et al. (1996) used GIS both to evaluate the risks of toxic spillage from road tankers carrying hazardous wastes and to devise routes which would minimise the risks of accidents. Similarly, Moore (1994) describes the use of GIS, linked to a dispersion model, as a basis for risk assessment of exposure to air pollution. Hopkinson et al. (1994) also outline the use of GIS as part of a decision support system for sustainable urban traffic planning, aimed at minimising social, health and environmental impacts.

Despite these examples, it remains clear that the real potential of GIS in the analysis of health data has yet to be fully exploited; compared to other areas of application, adoption of GIS in the health context has been relatively slow. A number of factors has probably contributed to this situation. One has been the relatively weak links which have traditionally existed between epidemiologists and geographers. Another, as noted earlier, has been the limited statistical capability of most proprietary GIS (Bailey, 1995). This has meant that most advanced statistical investigation has had to be conducted externally — an approach which, in the past, has been hindered by difficulties of data transfer into and out of GIS.

Many of these barriers are beginning to be overcome. By providing a common platform for investigation, GIS should help to strengthen the relationships between epidemiologists and geographers. While the statistical capability of most GIS is gradually being improved, however, there remains an argument that the transparency and user-controllability of many of the more advanced techniques (e.g. kriging) are still poor. System architecture in GIS is also becoming considerably more open, and dynamic links have been developed with a number of statistical packages. Rowlingson and Diggle (1991), for example, have developed a set of S-plus functions which provide an interactive link between ArcInto and S-Plus. For the future, therefore, it may be expected that GIS will play an increasingly important role in the small-area analysis of health data. Equally, it is important to continue to understand the limitations as well as the strengths of the approach, to avoid over- or mis-interpretation of spatial analysis of health data.

CLUSTER INVESTIGATION

Cluster investigation is an area of work that is increasingly involving the public health physician. A putative disease cluster may first be identified by concerned members of the public, be reported by the media, or perhaps come to light following concerns about a pollution source in the vicinity. In any event, the local public health department often finds itself compelled to respond, if only to allay public anxiety. Note that as areas at apparent 'low' risk do not come to the attention of the authorities, there is built in bias towards reporting disease excess.

Often reassurance is all that is required, since as noted above, for rare diseases in small areas, an apparent disease excess may depend crucially on only one or two cases — and these may not stand detailed scrutiny during an initial case-by-case review (Centers for Disease Control, 1990). Such a review deals only with the numerator (cases) of the risk estimate, whereas a proper epidemiological enquiry is concerned also with the denominator (population). The next steps will therefore usually involve identification of a population at risk and specification of a time frame so that disease rates can be calculated. Decisions taken at this stage may be critical as apparent 'clusters' may depend crucially on the boundaries chosen in time or space: 'The more narrowly the underlying population is defined, the less will be the number of expected cases, the greater will be the estimate of the excess rate, and often the more pronounced will be the statistical significance' (Olsen *et al.*, 1996).

Additionally, if an apparent 'cluster' of cases is subsequently linked to a pollution source, statistical testing is formally invalidated because of the post hoc nature of the observation. None the less, despite the potential for bias toward elevated rates, the observed/expected ratio may be close to one. Where further investigation is indicated, this should preferably be done for an independent time period or in a different geographic area exposed to a similar pollution source.

The Problem of Confounding

One major difficulty in interpretation is the issue of socio-economic confounding. Sources of pollution tend to be in socio-economically disadvantaged areas, while deprivation itself is strongly linked to ill-health and health-defining behaviour such as smoking. Failure to account for social deprivation could therefore seriously bias investigation of environmental risk factors and ill-health.

This potential for bias is illustrated by the results of a national study of cancer risk near municipal solid waste incinerators mentioned above (Elliott et al., 1996). Excess risk was reported for a number of cancer sites, including those strongly linked to deprivation such as stomach and lung. The excess persisted even after adjustment for deprivation measured at the small-area scale. In those areas with available data, an excess of similar size was also found for these and some other cancers during the period before the incinerators were operational, indicating the presence of residual confounding: incineration per se did not seem a likely explanation for the excess (Elliott et al., 1996).

DISEASE MAPPING

As well as the investigation of disease clusters, public health physicians are becoming increasingly involved in disease mapping. The maps are used mainly as a descriptive tool as they provide a succinct and visually appealing summary of complex geographical information. They are also used for surveillance to highlight areas at high risk and to aid policy formation and resource allocation. Encouraged perhaps by the ease of production, disease maps now appear routinely in many district public health reports in the UK. A map showing large swathes of 'red' (i.e. high) areas may have great impact on public opinion and policy makers! Unfortunately, naïve use of such methods shares many of the problems of cluster detection noted previously. These include distinguishing 'true' from apparent areas of disease excess, and dealing appropriately with the play of chance including the problem of multiple significance testing. Problems are most evident in small-area disease mapping since numbers of cases tend to be small and apparent large variability across the map may merely reflect random variation. Specifically, large sparsely populated areas with few cases may predominate.

Methods based on Bayesian statistics have been used to help remove the random component from the map (Clayton & Bernardinelli, 1992). An example is given in Fig. 7.1. It shows a map of 'unsmoothed' (standardised incidence ratio, adjusted for age, sex and deprivation) and smoothed (empirical Bayes) estimates of brain cancer incidence for 1974–86 across electoral wards in the West Midlands region of England (Eaton *et al.*, 1997). As can be seen, much of the random variability is removed by smoothing, especially the apparent high rates found in the large, sparsely populated rural areas. Overall, there is only weak evidence of heterogeneity across the map, $p = 0.04$ using the Potthoff–Whittinghill test (Eaton *et al.*, 1997; and see Alexander & Cuzick, 1992 for a description of the statistical method).

SMALL AREA GEOGRAPHIC CORRELATION STUDIES OF ENVIRONMENT AND HEALTH

As noted above, not only are health and population data used in geographic analyses, but also increasingly a range of environmental data are available as well. This raises the possibility of correlating the health and environmental data, for example within a GIS. Again, although intuitively attractive, this approach has many pitfalls for the unwary as there are major potential problems of ecological confounding and bias (the 'ecological fallacy') which could seriously distort the results of such investigations (English, 1992). None the less, carefully conducted small-area studies may be less prone to such biases as the level of analysis is closer to the individual than in traditional ecological studies. Indeed, an individual-level study can be thought of as an extreme example of an ecological study in which each 'cell' has either zero or one case!

Small Area Variations in Air Quality and Health – The SAVIAH study

The European Union funded SAVIAH study is a recent example of

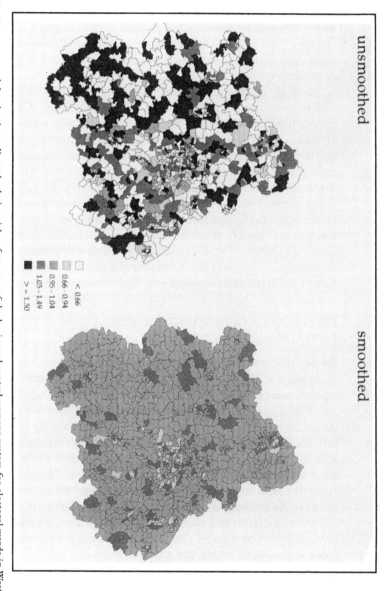

Fig. 7.1 Age-, sex- and deprivation adjusted relative risks of cancers of the brain and central nervous system for electoral wards in West Midlands region, England, age 15–64 years, 1974–86. Unsmoothed risks (left) and after map smoothing (right) using empirical Bayes method (from Eaton *et al.*, 1997 with permission.)

unsmoothed

smoothed

■ < 0.66
▨ 0.66 - 0.94
▧ 0.95 - 1.04
▨ 1.05 - 1.49
□ > = 1.50

a small-area study that examined both health effects (childhood symptoms of wheeze and cough) and environmental exposures (outdoor air pollution). Despite the major improvements in air quality which have been achieved in Britain over the last 30 years, the problem of air pollution and health remains a major public and policy concern. A large number of studies, mainly in the USA but also, increasingly, in Britain and the rest of Europe, have tended to demonstrate raised levels of respiratory morbidity and mortality associated with acute exposures to increased levels of air pollution, especially fine particulates and sulphur dioxide (for reviews, see Schwartz, 1994a,b; Committee on the Medical Effects of Air Pollution, 1995; Committee of the Environmental and Occupational Health Assembly of the American Thoracic Society, 1996). The potentially much larger impacts of chronic exposures to relatively low levels of air pollution (especially from traffic) have, in contrast, been less intensively studied and have proved to be more difficult to detect. One reason for this has been the comparatively poor development of the spatial analytical methods necessary to investigate such effects at the small-area scale.

The SAVIAH study employed a combination of questionnaire surveys, low-cost pollution monitoring, pollution modelling and small area statistical techniques, brought together within a GIS environment. The study was undertaken in four European cities: Huddersfield (UK), Amsterdam (Netherlands), Prague (Czech Republic) and Poznan (Poland). Details of the study are provided by Elliott *et al.* (submitted), Briggs *et al.* (1997), Lebret *et al.* (1997) and van Reeuwijk *et al.* (1997).

Health survey

In each centre, a survey was carried out of all children living and going to school within the study areas, using questionnaires delivered to parents and guardians. Age of the children ranged from 7–8 in Poznan to 7–11 in Amsterdam. In three of the centres, questionnaires were distributed through the schools; these all produced high response rates (88 – 96%). In the fourth area (Amsterdam), the questionnaires were delivered direct to the home (63% response rate). Questionnaires included a series of questions relating to personal and familial characteristics, domestic factors (e.g. smoking in the home, heating, presence of pets) and symptoms and diagnosis of asthma and wheeze, both within the last 12 months and over the lifetime of the child (ever). Results of the health survey showed some variability in apparent levels of morbidity in the four centres. The crude prevalence of wheeze-ever ranged from 22.8% in Amsterdam to 30% in Huddersfield, while rates of wheeze in the last 12 months varied from 10.2% in Amsterdam to 17.8% in Huddersfield. Prevalence was higher amongst boys than girls, in all centres.

Air pollution monitoring

To provide measures of exposure to outdoor air pollution, monitoring was conducted in each of the study areas using passive diffusion tubes (van Reeuwijk *et al.*, 1997). In three of the study areas (Huddersfield, Amsterdam, Prague), attention was focused on nitrogen dioxide as a proxy for exposure to traffic-related pollution; in Poznan, where the main source of emission was district heating plants, the focus was on sulphur dioxide. Four two-week sampling campaigns were carried out over a period of one year, two duplicate tubes being deployed at a series of 80 'permanent' sites on each occasion. Forty 'variable' sites were also measured on each occasion, these being relocated for each survey in order to examine different aspects of local variation. In addition, ten sites were monitored on a continuous basis in each study area, using tubes exposed for four-week periods (two-weeks during the main survey campaigns) in order to provide an independent estimate of the mean annual concentration. A mixed-effect analysis of variance model was applied to results from the 80 'permanent' sites for the four survey campaigns, with terms for measurement error and site-survey effects. This demonstrated systematic between-site variation in NO_2 levels across the study areas, accounting for 60–80% of the total variation (Lebret *et al.*, 1997).

GIS development

A geographical information system was built for each study area, using ArcInfo. Each GIS included relevant spatial and attribute information. Key data sets included:

- emission sources, (e.g. road network, traffic volume);
- land cover/land use;
- altitude;
- school locations and catchment areas;
- population distribution;
- small-area administrative boundaries, (e.g. enumeration districts, wards);

- location of surveyed children (in the UK, the centroid of the unit postcode of residence);
- pollution monitoring sites and concentrations.

Exposure assessment

Pollution maps were computed for each study area using a range of methods, including spatial interpolation (ordinary kriging) dispersion modelling and regression-mapping techniques. Validity of the maps was tested by comparing the predicted concentrations with the measured concentrations at the continuous sampling sites. Regression mapping consistently out-performed other methods, explaining 79–87% of the measured variation at the continuous sites, and was therefore used for subsequent mapping. Regression equations were constructed for each area by comparing measured pollution levels at the 80 'permanent' sites with a variety of predictor variables for a 300-metre buffer around the site, including measures of traffic volume, altitude and land cover (Briggs *et al.*, 1997). These equations were then applied to the whole study area, by passing a moving window across the map, and calculating the pollution level for each map pixel. Estimates of exposure to outdoor air pollution were then made for each respondent in the health survey by dropping a point on to the pollution map for the place of residence.

Health mapping

Results for the respiratory end points (cough and wheeze in last 12 months and ever) were mapped at the small-area scale to investigate the extent of spatial variation in health outcome. Map smoothing was carried out, using a simple Bayesian approach, based on the binomial distribution (Martuzzi & Elliott, 1996). Resulting patterns were tested for heterogeneity and spatial autocorrelation using the Potthoff–Whittinghill test and Moran statistic. Mostly, only the map for Huddersfield showed evidence of heterogeneity in respiratory symptom prevalence at the small-area level.

Relationships between outdoor air pollution and respiratory health

Relationships between predicted outdoor air pollution at residence of the child and respiratory symptoms were analysed using logistic regression, with control for potential confounding at individual level. No significant associations were found. This is consistent with the results of some studies of traffic-related pollution and asthma (Livingstone *et al.*, 1996) but not with others (Edwards *et al.*, 1994); such differences need to be reconciled, although the evidence to date does not indicate a strong effect of outdoor air pollution on asthma prevalence (Committee on Medical Effects of Air Pollutants, 1995). The SAVIAH study was primarily a methodological investigation, aimed at developing and testing small-area spatial techniques for analysing patterns of, and relationships between, air pollution and respiratory health. As such, it illustrates a number of methodological advances that have been made in recent years, especially in the area of pollution monitoring, GIS and small-area statistical techniques. These offer considerable scope for further development and application in other small-area studies of environmental pollution and health.

SUMMARY

The investment in large geo-referenced health datasets, the increasing availability of relevant environmental data, together with developments in computing, statistical methodologies and GIS have meant that sophisticated small-area analyses of health and environment are now possible at reasonable cost. It can be expected that such analyses will become increasingly prevalent in the future, not least because of the instant visual appeal offered by the new geographic techniques and their wide availability. However, if geographical analyses are to maintain scientific credibility, it is important that they are guided by good questions, sound epidemiological principles and excellent statistical methodology, while interpretation will need to take account of problems of data quality, completeness, bias and confounding. As the data and methodologies improve, it is to be expected that results of small-area studies will continue to contribute importantly to our understanding of the relationships between environment and health.

ACKNOWLEDGEMENTS

We are grateful to Ann Gould (Information and Statistics Division of the National Health Service in Scotland) for providing details of availability of Scottish data.

REFERENCES

Alexander FE, Boyle P, eds. 1996 Methods for investigating localised clustering of disease. Lyon, IARC Scientific Publications No. 135

Alexander F, Cuzick J 1992 Methods for the assessment of disease clusters. In Elliott P, Cuzick J, English D et al, eds. Geographical and Environmental Epidemiology: Methods for Small Area Studies. Oxford University Press, Oxford. pp.221–30

Bailey TC 1995 A review of statistical spatial analysis in geographical information systems. In Spatial Analysis and GIS. Fotheringham S, Rogerson P eds. London: Taylor and Francis, pp 13–44

Black D (chairman) 1984 Investigation of the Possible Increased Incidence of Cancer in West Cumbria. Report of the Independent Advisory Group. London: HMSO

Bower JS, Vallence-Plews J 1995 The UK national air monitoring networks. A talk for a WHO seminar, 21–23 November 1995. AEA Technology

Brainard J, Lovett A, Parfitt J 1996 Assessing hazardous waste transport risks using a GIS. International Journal of Geographical Information Systems 10 (7): 831–49

Briggs DJ 1995 Environmental statistics for environmental policy: genealogy and data quality. Journal of Environmental Management 44: 39–54

Briggs DJ, Elliott P 1995 GIS methods for the analysis of relationships between environment and health. World Health Statistics Quarterly 48: 85–94

Briggs DJ, Collins S, Elliott P, Kingham S, Fischer P, Lebret W, van Reeuwijk H, van der Veen A, Pryl K, Smallbone K 1997 Mapping urban air pollution using GIS: a regression-based approach. International Journal of Geographical Information Science (in press)

Campbell GW, Stedman J R, Stevenson K 1994 A survey of nitrogen dioxide concentrations in the United Kingdom using diffusion tubes July – December 1991. Atmospheric Environment 28(3): 477–87

Centers for Disease Control 1990. Guidelines for investigating clusters of health events. Mortality and Morbidity Weekly Report 39: (No. RR-11), 1–23

Clayton DG, Bernardinelli L 1992 In Geographical and Environmental Epidemiology: Methods for small-area studies, Elliott P, Cuzick J, English D, Stern R eds. Oxford University Press, Oxford, pp 205–220

Committee of the Environmental and Occupational Health Assembly of the American Thoracic Society 1996 Health effects of outdoor pollution. American Journal of Respiratory Critical Care Medicine 153, 3–50

Committee on Medical Effects of Air Pollutants 1995 Asthma and Outdoor Air Pollution. HMSO, London

Cuzick J, Elliott P 1992 Small-area studies: purpose and methods. In Geographical and Environmental Epidemiology: Methods for small-area studies, Elliott P, Cuzick J, English D, Stern R eds. Oxford University Press, Oxford, pp 14–21

Department of Environment 1996 Digest of Environmental Protection and Water Statistics, 1994. HMSO, London

Diamond I 1992 Population counts in small areas. In Geographical and Environmental Epidemiology: Methods for small-area studies, Elliott P, Cuzick J, English D, Stern R eds. Oxford University Press, Oxford, pp. 96–105

Dolk H, Elliott P, Shaddick G, Walls P, Thakrar B 1997a Cancer incidence near radio and television transmitters in Great Britain. II. All high power transmitters. American Journal of Epidemiology 145: 10–17

Dolk H, Shaddick G, Walls P, Grundy C, Thakrar B, Kleinschmidt I, Elliott P 1997b. Cancer incidence near radio and television transmitters in Great Britain. I. Sutton Coldfield transmitter. American Journal of Epidemiology 145: 1–9

Eaton N, Shaddick G, Dolk H, Elliott P 1997 Small-area study of the incidence of neoplasms of the brain and central nervous system among adults in the West Midlands Region, 1974–86. British Journal of Cancer 75 (7), 1080–83

Edwards J, Walters S, Griffiths RC 1994 Hospital admissions for asthma in preschool children: relationship to major roads in Birmingham, UK. Archives of Environmental Health 49: 223–7

Elliott P, Briggs D, Lebret E, Gorynski P, Kriz B. (submitted) Small area variations in air quality and health (SAVIAH study): relationship of childhood respiratory wheeze to road traffic pollution.

Elliott P, Martuzzi M, Shaddick G 1995 Spatial statistical methods in environmental epidemiology: a critique. Statistical Methods in Medical Research 4: 139–61

Elliott P, Shaddick G, Kleinschmidt I, Jolley D, Wals P, Beresford J, Grundy C 1996 Cancer incidence near municipal solid waste incinerators in Great Britain. British Journal of Cancer 73: 702–10

English D 1992 Geographical epidemiology and ecological studies. In Geographical and Environmental Epidemiology: Methods for small-area studies, Elliott P, Cuzick J, English D, Stern R eds. Oxford University Press, Oxford, pp 3–13

Gatrell A, Dunn CE 1994 GIS and spatial epidemiology: modelling the possible association between cancer of the larynx and incineration in North-West England. In The Added Value of Geographical Information Systems in Public and Environmental Health. de Lepper M J C, Scholten H C, Stern R M eds. Kluwer Academic Publications, Dordrecht, pp 215–35

Gatrell A, Rowlingson B 1995 Spatial point process modelling in a GIS environment. In Spatial Analysis and GIS. Fotheringham S, Rogerson P eds. Taylor and Francis, London, pp 147–63

Gatrell A, Mitchell JD, Gibson HN, Diggle PJ 1991 Tests for spatial clustering in epidemiology: with special reference to Motor Neurone Disease. In New Evidence in MND/ALS Research. Rose C ed. Smith-Gordon and Company, London

Glass GE, Schwartz BS, Morgan JM, Johnson DT, Noy PM, Israel E 1995 Environmental risk factors for lyme disease identified with geographic information systems. American Journal of Public Health 85(7): 944–8

Hopkinson P, Webber P, Briggs DJ 1994 Developing an environmental management system for traffic pollution impacts. Transportation Planning Systems 2: 39–52

Langford M, Maguire DJ, Unwin DJ 1991 The area interpolation problem: estimating population using remote sensing in a GIS framework. In Handling Geographical Information: Methodology and Potential Applications. Masser I, Blakemore M eds. Longman Scientific and Technical, London, pp 55–77

Lebret E, Briggs D, Collins S, van Reeuwijk H, Fischer P, Harssema H, Kriz B, Gorynski P, Elliott P 1997 Small area variations in ambient NO_2 exposures in four European areas: the SAVIAH study. Atmospheric Environment (in press)

Lefohn AS, Knudsen HP, McEvoy LR 1988 The use of kriging to estimate monthly ozone exposure parameters for the southeastern United States. Environmental Pollution 53: 27–42

Liu LJS, Rossini A, Koutrakis P 1995 Development of cokriging models to predict 1- and 12-hour ozone concentrations in Toronto. (Abstract). Epidemiology 6(4): S69

Livingstone AE, Shaddick G, Grundy C, Elliott P 1996 Do people living near inner city main roads have more asthma needing treatment? Case-control study. British Medical Journal 312: 676–7

Martuzzi M, Elliott P 1996 Empirical Bayes estimation of small area prevalence of non-rare conditions. Statistics in Medicine 15: 1867–73

Moore TJ 1994 The potential role of geographical information systems technology in air toxics risk assessment, communication and management. In The Added Value of Geographical Information Systems in Public and Environmental Health. de Lepper MJC, Scholten HC, Stern RM eds. Kluwer Academic Publications, Dordrecht, pp 237–62

Noy D, Brunekreef B, Boliej JSM, Houthuijs D, Koning de R 1990 The assessment of personal exposure to nitrogen dioxide in epidemiological studies. Atmospheric Environment 24A: 2903–9

Oliver MA, Webster R 1990 Kriging: a method of interpolation for geographical information systems. International Journal of Geographical Information Systems 4: 313–32

Olsen SF, Martuzzi M, Elliott P 1996 Cluster analysis and disease mapping — why, when, and how? A step by step guide. British Medical Journal 313: 863–86

Openshaw S Charlton M, Wymer C, Craft AW, 1987 A mark 1 Geographical Analysis Machine for the automated analysis of point data sets. International Journal of Geographical Information Systems 1: 335–58

Openshaw S, Cross A, Charlton M, 1990 Building a prototype Geographical Correlates Exploration Machine. International Journal of Geographical Information Systems 4 (3): 297–312

Rowlingson B, Diggle PJ 1991 SPLANCS: spatial point pattern analysis code in S-plus. Computers and Geosciences 19: 627–55

Schwartz J 1994a Air pollution and daily mortality: a review and meta-analysis. Environmental Research 64: 36–52

Schwartz J 1994b What are people dying of on high air pollution days. Environmental Research 64: 26–35

Stein A, Staritsky I, Bouma J, van Groenigen JW 1995 Interactive GIS for environmental risk assessment. International Journal of Geographical Information Systems 9(5): 509–25

van Reeuwijk H, Fischer P, Harsemma H, Briggs DJ, Smallbone K, Lebret E 1997 Field comparison of two NO_2 passive samplers to assess spatial variation. Environmental Monitoring and Assessment (in press)

Vincent P, Gatrell A 1991 The spatial distribution of radon gas in Lancashire (UK): a kriging study. In Proceedings of the Second European Conference on Geographical Information Systems. EGIS Foundation, Utrecht, pp 1179–86

Wartenberg D 1993 Some epidemiologic applications of kriging. In Geostatistics Troia '92. Vol 2. Soares A ed. Kluwer, Quantitative Geology and Statistics 5, New York, pp 911–22

Wilkinson P, Elliott P, Grundy C, Shaddick G, Thakrar B, Walls P, Falconer S 1997a Case-control study of hospital admission with asthma in children aged 5–14 years: relation with road traffic in North West London. *Thorax* (in press)

Wilkinson P, Thakrar B, Shaddick G, Stevenson S, Pattenden S, Landon M, Grundy C, Elliott P 1997b Cancer incidence and mortality around the Pan Britannica Industries pesticide factory, Waltham Abbey. Occupational and Environmental Medicine 54: 101–7

Williams ML 1995 Monitoring of exposure to air pollution. The Science of the Total Environment 168: 169–74

8. Community Development and Social Deprivation

Gina Radford, Debra Lapthorne, Neil Boot, and Moira Maconachie

INTRODUCTION

Living, socialising, educating, growing, developing, being and dying have to be authentically our own experience. What neutralises and disempowers both individuals and communities is being denied the opportunity of being what they want to be and what they know they can be.

(Jones P, Presentation to the Healthy Plymouth Conference 1993)

This chapter presents two perspectives of the role of community development. The first suggests it is an essential development if we are to maximise health gain. The second section suggests a degree of caution is necessary before the approach is wholeheartedly embraced.

COMMUNITY DEVELOPMENT AND PUBLIC HEALTH

It may be suggested that community development and public health share common roots in that they have both sought to change the determinants of health through collective or population based action. They both seek to influence a wide variety of agencies to bring about change which will impact upon the health of a local or wider population. They both belong to what Smithies (1991: 25) describes as the 'community health movement' in that they are part of a 'loosely defined social movement' which recognises that dynamic change in the health status of a population needs 'collective tactics and strategies' not just single agency action.

Community development and public health may seem to present polarised views of this social movement but this section will set out some of the reasons why closer partnerships between the two has the potential for significant gain. Community development is a process by which people are involved in collectively defining and taking action on issues that affect their lives. It seeks to enable communities to grow and change according to their own needs and priorities. Community development for health is the application of community development principles and practices to the health context. Community development for health is not a new phenomenon; initiatives such as the Peckham Project which sought to tackle the root causes of ill health as well as delivering a traditional medical response to its effects, predate the NHS.

Community development for health describes the process of stimulating the participation of local communities in bringing about improvements in health. Participation can take different forms but is established as a core principle of the approach. Communities can be geographical such as a neighbourhood or describe a community of interest like older people, but the method is usually applied in areas where communities experience material or social deprivation. Communities such as these usually experience the poorest health (Benzeval *et al.*, 1995).

HISTORICAL CONTEXT

Community development originated in the 1970s and has been linked to health work in many different ways since then, often as part of a wider social movement based on different issues such as gender or race. The politicisation of such issues in the past led to fears that working to local people's agendas often meant working against the statutory agencies, resulting in conflict. The current movement within community development is much more about negotiation and working together with agencies to achieve a common goal rather than being in conflict. Community development for health aims to develop structures which enable the active involvement of all in the promotion of community health. In order to do this it bases its work on a set of core values:

• Community participation and empowerment is essential to enable communities to have the opportunity, ability and confidence to fully participate in improving the health and well being of the communities in which they live and work;
• Work should be targeted at reducing variations in health;
• Partnership and collaboration between organisations is necessary in order to promote health and positive well being.

The bringing together of community members and professionals into 'health alliances' is a common feature of more recent community development initiatives. These alliances can act as a powerful force in bringing about change. Change is usually brought about by the community identifying and articulating their own health needs and agenda for action; starting and managing their own neighbourhood organisations and groups such as community businesses or setting up and running community facilities, events and activities like food or furniture co-operatives, play schemes and health fairs; campaigning or negotiating for improvements in the area (e.g. better play or leisure facilities, improved transport links, improvements to sub-standard housing) strengthening community networks, relationships and support, providing mutual aid for better health (e.g. parents' drug advice line, befriending schemes) promoting a stronger sense of community spirit, helping to foster people's sense of worth, identity and belonging, reducing isolation and feelings of helplessness; building self-esteem and personal skills (anticipating that this may lead to reductions in crime and improvements in mental health.)

At a wider strategic level, individual community developments can be aggregated across a district to point to defects in public policy and provision. There is wide recognition now that health is not just the responsibility of Health Authorities and many of the factors which impact upon people's health, such as housing, employment and the environment are part of a wider responsibility for many other agencies. Health is 'everyone's business'.

CHALLENGES

In the NHS there is an increased demand both for more resources and better use of the resources currently available. There is an increasing ageing population with many more people living well into their eighties and beyond. The poverty divide is getting wider, with the health gap between the richer and the poorer sections of our communities getting bigger. It is generally recognised that community development offers an effective way of addressing health variations (Benzeval et al., 1995).

Health Authorities also have a new enabling role, which is broader than just the purchasing of services, which builds on work already undertaken working together with local people to find solutions to their needs. Furthermore Public Health departments act as the gateway to enormous amounts of data about the impact of poverty upon health and are in an ideal position to share this with other agencies and community groups to help them determine their own priorities for action.

As Harrison (1996) notes, Health Authorities have responsibility for a number of functions, one of which, assessing the health needs of their local population, requires them to take into account the views expressed by local people. In order for this process to be meaningful, a way has to be found for local people to be involved in both identifying the needs as well as the development of a response to such needs. Community development offers such a mechanism to Health Authorities to enable them to do this.

Communities also need statutory agencies to consider how they will develop organisationally to engage meaningfully with communities and receive the information generated by local health needs assessment. Taylor (1996) describes this as 'working at the interface of two realities: the expectations of the organisation...and the reality and expectations of the local community'. The real challenge for statutory agencies such as Health Authorities in embracing community development is one of organisational development for without it the potential for significant health gain will not be realised. 'Any inequality in the availability and use of health services in relation to need is in itself socially unjust and requires alleviation' (Townsend & Davidson, 1982: 68).

People who are at the lower end of the socio-economic groupings, have less choice in every area of their lives. Physical and mental survival has to take precedence over health-enhancing activities. Community-led health initiatives to address health inequalities such as the Deprivation Initiative in Plymouth and the Stockport Health Promise combine a strategic response with practical support and are focused on some of the more basic needs of people to survive.

They are based on, and include, a community development approach as a way of addressing health inequalities and provide facilitation and support of local involvement. This approach moves away from a limited, more traditional approach which can encourage dependence upon professionals and often perpetuates 'victim blaming' as a reason for an inability to achieve health gain. They support practical schemes such as credit unions and food co-operatives which help to give people back a choice about what they would like to or can do by directly impacting upon poverty. They also work with local people to increase access to existing or develop more appropriate services. The value of approaches which perpetuate victim blaming are now more likely to be seen as of limited or no worth. Blaxter (1989) argues that 'if attention is concentrated on improving lifestyles, at the expense of action to diminish material deprivation, existing inequalities in health will widen even further.' Community development can offer a transferable model of identifying needs and gaps in service provision which also facilitates consumer involvement. The community development approach to health is positive and proactive and can enable people not only to access but also to develop more appropriate services.

Health gain can only be achieved through active partnership with local people and by the collective policy response to the realities of the impact of poverty upon people's lives. By embracing a community development approach to health the Public Health movement can support processes whereby communities and the individuals within them can be empowered to help themselves. This needs more than a co-ordinated government approach to the alleviation of poverty. There needs to be acknowledgement that health is not something that communities receive passively still less something that Health Authorities can purchase. Health, particularly the health of communities is something they are capable of helping to provide for themselves.

DIFFICULTIES ENCOUNTERED WITH COMMUNITY DEVELOPMENT APPROACHES

It is important to balance the promise of adopting a community development approach with a consideration of the practical problems that may be encountered in doing so. It is not uncommon for there to be a gap between the optimism of those who emphasise the advantages of an approach in order to persuade others of the merit of similarly adopting it, and the reality encountered in the field which can consist in rather more compromise than promise. Advocates of community development approaches are fortunate because community-based initiatives and local participation have gained popularity and among some supporters may be considered beyond question, as self-evidently good ideas. None the less, the intention in this section is to ask questions and to consider the difficulties associated with community development initiatives.

At the outset, it should be said that community development is not simple or easily done, and that the parameters of 'bottom-up' approaches are not always clear. The term 'community' provokes sceptics to enquire about what is meant by 'the community': who precisely does it include and exclude? Acknowledging that communities are not homogeneous, are to some degree 'imagined', is not enough to satisfy the curiosity of those who want to know how different experiences, diverse points of view and conflicting interests are identified and taken into account in the process of community development. They also remain doubtful about the normative elements suggested by the term 'community'. It is important to clarify early on whether or not it is possible to speak of 'the community' let alone on behalf of 'the community'. At stake are issues of inclusivity and coverage which also need to be considered in relation to claims made about accountability and democratisation. If the process of community development involves creating a forum or platform for putting forward community perspectives, how much confidence is there that the variety of possible perspectives will be represented? How reliable is the process? There is concern that community-based initiatives can become vehicles for particular interests and organised groups, and that those who are 'marginalised' may not be included and consequently not be heard.

Involving community members in identifying their health needs, in priority setting and in planning and evaluating services is regarded as an important challenge to the unequal relationships — relationships of power — that currently shape access to information, decision-making and funding. Community development approaches may reveal that a gap exists between professional and lay perspectives (in conceptualising, interpreting and understanding health issues) and that dialogue between the two is crucial for mutual understanding and appropriate planning to take place. Mikkelsen's (1995: 28) basic definition of participation is 'people deciding over their own lives'. Accepting this broad definition, there are different modes of participation including, 'Co-option, compliance, consultation, co-operation, co-learning, and collective action' (Mikkelsen, 1995: 96). What matters is the form and scope of the participation that occurs. And the question that arises concerns not only who is involved, but also the conditions on which they become involved and participate.

There are obstacles in the way of readily achieving 'open dialogue'. Professionals, experts and agency workers commonly find it hard to cede or hand over control and to share decision-making with others. Power is not often relinquished nor is control over policy usually abandoned by those who have it. Whether and how far decision-making is to be devolved to communities is likely to prove contentious. Does participation also entail accepting responsibility for any decisions made? How feasible or even desirable this would be from the point of view of community members is also questionable. It is not possible to just assume that members of communities are willing to become fully involved. It is possible, for example, that community members may welcome consultation without wanting to assume responsibility for final decision making.

Securing participation and involvement is likely to be time consuming for everyone, including community members. And sustaining the process of engagement is important so that expectations are not raised without a chance of some of them being met. Community development that is not initiated by community members but by outside agencies predictably raises ethical issues for the professionals who get involved (rights to confidentiality, to silence, to end participation, for example, are linked to concerns about social authoritarianism). In some circumstances, there is an additional danger that the boundaries between professional work and advocacy or activism might become confused. Community development initiatives are not ordinarily regarded as a substitute for or an alternative to local political processes and structures.

Community development approaches that are transformational (rather than merely instrumental) are concerned about empowerment (through participation, understanding local issues, acquiring skills and confidence), engagement and partnership working. Although empowerment cannot be 'delivered' (people are not empowered but rather empower themselves), the 'success' of community development initiatives (especially when initiated by outside agencies) depends to a large extent on the commitment and skills of the community development worker(s) involved. But the evaluation of success is difficult because it is not clear what criteria should be used to assess community development initiatives that are 'process oriented', especially in the short term. In areas where there is little sense of community, poor housing, high levels of unemployment and family breakdown, for example, what is expected of community development workers could be unrealistic. This is especially the case when short-term appointments are made and when both funding and support is limited. Adopting a community development approach is not a 'quick-fix' option.

Community development requires a long-term perspective and this makes the approach time-consuming, costly, and often difficult to evaluate. All of which can make it difficult to raise the levels of funding that are often required. Within a framework of limited resources and where there is the responsibility to allocate scarce resources equitably and in an accountable way, adopting a community-development approach is more difficult. The approach is said to be most appropriate in areas of social deprivation, but what criteria should be used to select a particular area or areas for long-term funding? Deprivation indices and scores could be used to rank areas, but different indices may produce different rankings. The Public Health Team in South & West Devon has examined the variation in how wards and 'neighbourhoods' are ranked depending on the measure of deprivation used (Nelder & Maconachie, 1997). The deprivation measures used (Breadline Britain, Townsend, Index of Local Conditions) and the Jarman Score produced different rankings. These differences are illustrated in Fig. 8.1 which shows the rankings of different wards for one locality within the Health Authority.

If deprivation indices are to be used to identify areas, it is not immediately apparent which measure of deprivation should be

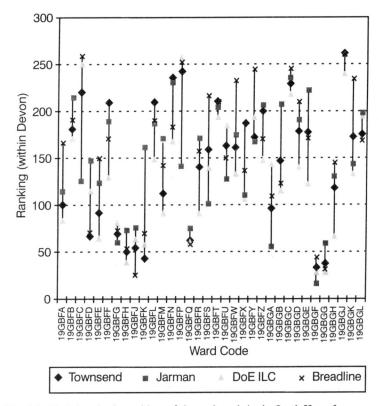

Fig. 8.1   Variations in the rankings of electoral wards in the South Hams for selected measures. (Produced by the Public Health Team, South and West Devon Health Authority, 1997.)

used. In addition to which measure to use, is the problem that the measures are based on census variables and cannot be updated between each census (every 10 years). More importantly, although these measures identify areas of relative deprivation it is also obvious that people who experience multiple deprivation also live in other areas and have legitimate claims. And it is not clear that committing long-term funding to a few selected areas only would necessarily be the most equitable and effective means of meeting the health needs of the many families and individuals who are living in poverty throughout South and West Devon. While sensitive to local community issues, public health has to maintain a broad and strategic perspective which addresses the health concerns of the whole population of the authority.

Community development has a local focus in its concern with particular areas or communities and in its emphasis on the contribution that 'bottom-up' approaches make to an understanding of public health issues. The final question of this discussion is to ask whether adopting a 'bottom-up' community development approach is by itself sufficient. The answer has to be negative. A public health perspective able to successfully link 'bottom-up' and 'top-down' approaches within a national and local framework is needed to meet the challenges posed by an expanding public health agenda.

CONCLUSION

This chapter has offered two versions on the role of community development and public health. It is clearly a valuable and exciting tool, and one that may help redress the traditional medical model of health, and balance the 'top-down' approach to needs assessment. However, as an approach it has limitations. Enthusiasts may claim it enables communities to identify and take action on issues to improve health. Sceptics may raise concerns about distinguishing needs and demands, about who really sets the agenda, and concerns about raising expectations unrealistically. However, community development is here to stay. The challenge is to ensure it is used appropriately and its limitations as well as its possibilities are recognised.

REFERENCES

Benzeval M, Judge K, Whitehead M 1995 Tackling Inequalities in Health: An Agenda for Action. King's Fund, London
Blaxter M 1989 A comparison of measures of inequality in morbidity. In: Health Inequalities in European Countries. Fox J ed. Gower, Aldershot

Harrison L 1996 Needs assessment and the National Health Service: context and change. In Identifying Local Health Needs, New Community Based Approaches. Burton P, Harrison L eds. The Policy Press, Bristol

Mikkelsen B 1995 Methods for Development Work and Research. Sage, New Delhi

Nelder R, Maconachie M 1997 Deprivation Scores at Electoral Ward Level within South & West Devon Health Authority (Information Document 1). South & West Devon Health Authority, Dartington

Smithies J 1991 A personal view of the history and current key issues and debates. In Community Development and Health: Reclaiming the National Agenda (Report of a National Seminar). The Public Health Alliance, Birmingham

Taylor P 1996 Supporting community involvement: the organisational challenges. In Identifying Local Health Needs, New Community Based Approaches. Burton P, Harrison L eds. The Policy Press, Bristol

Townsend P, Davidson N eds. 1982 Inequalities in Health: the Black Report. Penguin, Harmondsworth

9. Communicable Disease Challenges and Control

Patrick Wall and Rosalind Stanwell Smith

Infectious disease which antedated the emergence of human kind will last as long as humanity itself, and will surely remain, as it has been hitherto, one of the fundamental parameters and determinants of human history

(William McNeill, *Plagues and Peoples*, 1976)

INTRODUCTION

Once expected to be eliminated as a public health problem, infectious diseases remain the leading cause of death world-wide (WHO, 1992). Due to the inequitable distribution of the world's resources, some countries carry a disproportional heavy burden of infectious disease and what is considered a resurgent pathogen in one geographical location may be endemic in another. Historical successes in treating and controlling some of these diseases has left many health policy makers with the false perception that they no longer pose a threat to the public health in developed countries. In the second half of this century, public health practitioners have not so much neglected infection as to put it aside, in favour of more seemingly modern challenges. But infection is not easily marginalised and can, with ease, return to take the centre stage in public health. As things stand, infections continue to contribute significantly in terms of morbidity and increased costs of health care in developed countries.

The last two decades have presented several pressing infection problems, many of which are still current and are covered in this chapter. In several cases the solutions are known and the problem is to improve access, such as to vaccination or sanitation, or to change attitudes and mores, such as in hygiene practices and sexual behaviour. Familiarity with these problems, and a certain amount of apathy when progress seems painfully slow, has reduced the excitement that one associates with a new challenge. In identifying the important aspects of infection, we need to examine those which could excite new initiatives. A perception of changing challenge based on public health history is also helpful in selecting where priority should be placed. Using this approach, criteria can be devised to assess the degree of modern challenge. First, whether the history of the organism or disease has reached a crisis point, or a point at which action and new initiatives are urgent. Secondly, a technological criterion can be used: where new technology, such as new pharmaceuticals or electronic transmission of information exist, presenting the opportunity for control provides a feasible challenge. Thirdly, and not least, is the criterion of public perception and perceived need. We ignore the public interest in infections at our peril, as countless recent outbreaks testify. But the public factor is not restricted to the atavistic fear of contagion. The advance of science has raised expectations way beyond the challenges perceived by pioneers such as Louis Pasteur and John Snow in the 19th century. Expectations include longevity of life, safe travel and healthy children. Where infection abruptly disappoints these expectations, the public reaction is understandably one of anger and distrust for authority and those who purport to protect their health. The high expectations are not only those of the lay public: public health practitioners have also turned, with some relief, to other issues, covered elsewhere in this book. We constantly have to re-discover the threat of infection just because we share a deep need to feel we have not just colonised, but have conquered, the realm of the microbes.

The exact aetiology of many diseases is complex, or is not known, which makes control and prevention strategies difficult. However this is not true for most infectious diseases where prevention, control, containment or eradication is possible. In addition, increasing numbers of chronic diseases and cancers are been identified to have possible infectious aetiologies, presenting new opportunities for intervention. *Helicobacter pylori* infections are associated with peptic ulcer disease, papilloma virus type 16 with cervical cancer, hepatitis B and C with chronic liver disease and hepatocellular carcinoma and EB virus with lymphoma and nasopharyngeal tumours. *Chlamydia* infections have been tentatively linked with coronary artery disease and *Chlamydia pneumonia* has been grown from plaque material. Atheroma itself is in part an inflammatory process, and it is known only too well that microbes are excellent inducers of inflammation. Other diseases with possible infectious components in their aetiology include leukaemias, juvenile onset diabetes, multiple sclerosis, Kawasaki disease and Alzheimer disease (CDC, 1994).

EMERGING AND RE-EMERGING INFECTIONS

Emerging infectious diseases are diseases of infectious origin whose incidence in humans has increased within the past two decades or threatens to increase in the near future (Institute of Medicine, 1992). Examples of emerging infections include HIV/AIDS, verocytotoxin producing *Escherichia coli* O157, Cryptosporidiosis, legionnaires' disease, hepatitis C, *Vibrio cholerae* O139, etc. Re-emergence of infectious diseases may occur because of the development of antimicrobial resistance in existing agents (e.g. *Staphylococcus aureus*, *Neisseria gonorrhoeae*, *Streptococcus pneumonia*, *Mycobacterium* tuberculosis) or breakdown in public health measures for previously controlled infections (e.g. tuberculosis).

Many factors are contributing to the changing epidemiology of infectious diseases. An increasing proportion of the population of developed countries are elderly, and a growing number of persons are immune suppressed as a result of various medical interventions including organ and tissue transplants, cancer chemotherapy and other therapies causing immune suppression. Patients with HIV/AIDS are suffering from one infection, and the resultant immune suppression leaves them susceptible to many more. These immune suppressed individuals are at increased risk of infectious disease with devastating consequences and consume large amounts of costly health care resources. In addition, the increasing number of elderly people in residential care and policies of early discharge from hospital have resulted in large numbers of highly vulnerable individuals being cared for in the community setting where social and nursing care may not always be adequate. This permits infectious diseases to spread with ease. Economic necessity and social pressure for both parents to go out to work, and increasing numbers of single parent families, have resulted in many young children being placed in nurseries, presenting another opportunity for the spread of pathogens.

Many developing cities are growing so rapidly than their water supply and sewage treatment infrastructures are unable to keep pace and high morbidity and mortality from infectious diseases result, particularly in childhood. Intensive animal and poultry production units can produce an amount of effluent equivalent to a small town and it requires safe disposal. Environmental changes resulting from floods, droughts, famines, wars and civil unrest can present opportunities for infectious diseases to spread. Ease of modern travel has given infections unprecedented opportunity for spread across the world. While bacteria have benefited from these widened horizons, the largest new challenge comes from viruses, for example, imports of measles, influenza, and, via animal vectors, rabies. Geographers have vividly demonstrated the spatial dynamics of epidemics, for example in showing how the Influenza A pandemic of 1957/58 depended in part upon transmission via travellers on the Trans-Siberian Railway and sea routes, with a smaller contribution from air travel. Similarly, the upsurge in infectious diseases during the second World War, e.g. meningococcal meningitis, has been attributed to increased social mobility during this period. The implications of the enormous increase in air travel for infection spread are obvious and of particular concern with the potential for drift and shift of strains of Influenza A.

Transmission of infections within aircraft and ships is now well established, e.g. for tuberculosis, and these vehicles can also carry other unwanted passengers such as mosquitoes, bringing the possibility of malaria spread to previously cleared zones. In the UK, malaria is becoming increasingly common in returning holidaymakers, and the recent Ebola outbreaks emphasise that the possibility exists that more sinister infections may arrive on our doorstep. Travel-acquired infection is thus no longer merely an issue for long-haul travellers or the temporary irritation of travellers' diarrhoea. Increasing international travel has contributed to the introduction and dissemination of new pathogens. Once cholera had reached Peru in 1991, it rapidly spread across the Americas in months. Inadequate sanitation, as well as rapid travel of goods and people, will have played an important part in this event. In addition, tourists can return home with exotic infections.

The public health challenge is immense: it is unlikely that increased social mobility or frequent foreign travel will be reversed; it is predicted to continue to rise. We have the technology to rapidly inform other countries of episodes and trends in infectious diseases. But, there are still considerable political difficulties in ensuring early and honest notification of disease risks to other countries. With some infections, such as influenza, even early warning may not be soon enough to provide the time to develop appropriate vaccines. Perhaps one of the public health contributions will be to address the third factor, that of public awareness. In contrast to the fear in the past of importing infections, the very fear that led to quarantine regulations in Italy in the 14th century and to the self-sacrificing isolation of the Derbyshire plague village, Eyam, there is an expectation that travel-related disease is readily avoidable or at least treatable. Draconian preventive measures, such as barriers to travel, quarantine or compulsory immunisation of new arrivals are not well received. When insecticide sprays are used on aeroplanes, there is frequently an outcry from the passengers. The travel industry is well aware of the commercial sensitivity of infection and of the rapid effect that public fear can have on bookings: it is unlikely that major initiatives on limiting infection spread will come from this quarter. The long-awaited revision of public health legislation could provide an opportunity for improved monitoring of imported disease; communicable disease surveillance could also make a more focused contribution to measuring the extent of travel-related infection, whether from travel at home or abroad.

Advances in medicine are resulting in an increasing number of organ and tissue transplants, with xenotransplants on the horizon creating the potential for transfer of animal pathogens to hosts immune suppressed to prevent graft rejection.

FOOD AND WATERBORNE DISEASE

Infections transmitted by food and public water supplies place entire communities at risk and a succession of well publicised scares, e.g. *Salmonella* in eggs, *Listeria* in soft cheeses and pâté, *Campylobacter* in poultry and VTEC O157 and BSE in beef have shaken consumer confidence in the microbiological safety of food. Eating habits, especially in industrialised countries, are changing rapidly. There is an increasing tendency for people to eat more meals outside the home, to buy food in bulk (and less often) and to eat more 'fast foods' which require less preparation. Increasing mass production and global distribution of ready-to-eat foods present the opportunity for the dissemination of emerging or re-emerging infections, and put large populations at risk. Intensive farming of animals, poultry and fish facilitates the transmission of pathogens within the reservoir of human zoonotic infections. At all stages from the producer to the consumer, increased awareness of food hygiene is necessary to avoid extensive outbreaks. International surveillance is necessary if infections related to the global distribution of food are to be identified and controlled. Salm-Net is a developing system for the surveillance of salmonellosis in Europe, but has also been used successfully for other pathogens. With its links within the European Union and its extended links to parallel electronic and manual reporting systems in other surveillance centres outside Europe, it has demonstrated its usefulness in the rapid identification of outbreaks and enabled the early introduction of control measures.

In 1994 Salm-Net was successfully used to identify and enable rapid control of an international outbreak of *Shigella* dysentery in three European countries associated with the consumption of iceberg lettuce exported from a fourth. In 1995, Salm-Net aided in the investigation of a cluster of cases of *S. agona* in England, associated with the consumption of a peanut-flavoured snack which led to the recognition and control of outbreaks in Canada and the USA and a massive outbreak involving over 2000 cases in Israel. The identification of a contaminated product with a widespread distribution demonstrates the benefits of international surveillance and collaborative investigation. Competition in the food industry may force manufacturers to put cost reduction before food safety, therefore it is important that retailers make food safety a top priority so that companies compete on that basis. It is unrealistic to assume that all microbiological hazards can be eliminated; therefore, efforts must be directed to reduce their occurrence as far as possible. The focus must be on limiting the growth, survival and spread of pathogens in foodstuffs and, considering the susceptibility of the particular consumers, agreements should be reached on what levels of these pathogens are acceptable in which foods.

Campylobacter and *Salmonella* account for most of the laboratory reports and probably also of food poisoning notifications. The importance of *Campylobacter* as a human pathogen was recognised in the late 1970s and it is now the commonest gastrointestinal pathogen isolated from human beings in the UK. There is a characteristic seasonal distribution of reports, with a peak in the early summer, in contrast to reports of salmonella which reach their maximum in the late summer and autumn. There are also regional variations in the reporting of *Campylobacter* infections, which may reflect a higher incidence in rural than urban populations. The vast majority of cases are sporadic and may be associated with the consumption of poultry. *Campylobacter* do not multiply in food and most of the larger outbreaks are due to the consumption of unpasteurised milk or water contaminated with animal faeces. Cases have been associated with the consumption of milk from bottles where the tops have been pecked by birds, who are believed to transfer infection on their beaks from animal faeces upon which they have previously been feeding.

Salmonella continues to be one of the main causes of foodborne illness world-wide: the organism is ubiquitous among domestic and wild, warm-blooded, animals and avian species. One feature of salmonella is their ability to adapt to different species and to take advantage of changing environmental factors. Although there are more than 2200 serovars of *Salmonella*, *S. enteritidis* and *S. typhimurium* account for three-quarters of reported cases in the Great Britain, where there has been a dramatic increase in salmonellosis since 1984. This increase has been almost entirely due to *S. enteritidis*, particulary PT4. The intensive rearing of poultry using strains of poultry selected for food conversion efficiency and egg production rather than disease resistance provided fertile ground for *S. enteritidis*. *S. enteritidis* PT4 causes an invasive infection in poultry that leads to septicaemia and subsequent chronic infection of various organs; when the ovary is infected transmission of the organisms to the contents of the egg can occur. Contamination of eggs and poultry meat and an increasing consumption of poultry meat has led to the predominance of *S. enteritidis* PT4 as a cause of human salmonellosis. Various European countries have also experienced a higher incidence of *S. enteritidis* PT4 infections, and the organism has been isolated from human cases and food items from over ten European countries and from countries as far apart as the USA, Argentina and Japan. Since 1990, in the UK, there has been a dramatic increase in multidrug resistant *S. typhimurium* DT104 and this strain is now the second most common cause of salmonella food poisoning after *S. enteritidis* PT4. It is a cause of disease in cattle, sheep, pigs and poultry, and this wide food animal reservoir enables a diverse range of foodstuffs to become contaminated. *S. enteritidis* PT4 is primarily a problem with poultry meat and eggs yet has proved extremely difficult to control. Therefore, *S. typhimurium* DT104 with its diverse animal reservoir presents a formidable challenge to public health professionals, veterinarians, farmers and the food industry.

Among the enterovirulent *E. coli*, verocytoxin producing enterohaemorrhagic *E coli* O157 has emerged as a public health problem(EHEC). It was first identified as a human pathogen in the USA in 1982 Although the actual numbers of cases in the UK are small, it is of concern because of its serious complications, haemorrhagic colitis and haemolytic uraemic syndrome, and its high mortality rate. An outbreak in Lanarkshire in Scotland in 1996 resulted in over 400 affected people and 20 deaths, demonstrating that we become complacent about the safety of food at our peril.

In the spring of 1993, contamination of a municipal water supply with the intestinal parasite *Cryptosporidium parvum* caused a massive outbreak of waterborne illness in the United States. An estimated 403,000 persons in Milwaukee, Wisconsin, had prolonged diarrhoea; approximately 4400 persons required hospitalisation and 100 people died. Following a large waterborne outbreak of cryptosporidiosis in England in 1989, a government committee was convened which produced two reports containing a series of recommendations (Badenoch 1 and 2 (1990, 1995)). However, outbreaks continue to occur and one involving 500 confirmed cases occurred in the Torbay area in 1995. Therefore, in 1997 in the UK we cannot take access to potable water for granted and adequate surveillance is necessary to rapidly detect outbreaks. Chlorination does not destroy Cryptosporidium and the potential for widespread dissemination exists.

GENETICALLY ENGINEERED FOOD

Foodstuffs have been genetically engineering to increase their shelf-life or make them resistant to herbicides or particular pests. Often an antibiotic resistance gene is also inserted and used as a marker to indicate that the genetic modification is present. Fears exist that these antibiotic resistance genes could transfer to bacteria in the gastrointestinal tracts of animals or humans. Consumers should be free to choose non-genetically modified food, and their freedom depends on accurate labelling.

NEW VARIANT CJD AND BSE

The magnitude of the present epidemic of bovine spongiform encephalopathy (BSE) is without precedent in the recorded history of the transmissible spongiform encephalopathies. The public health and the scientific issues have become entwined in the political and commercial response to increasing national and international concern over the possibility of transmission of spongiform encephalopathy from cattle to man. Public health professionals must respond to the intense public anxiety regarding the risk to the nation of exposure to BSE-contaminated material. Documented transmission of BSE to non-human primates indicates that such anxiety is not without scientific foundation. We are left facing possible present consequences of past events over which we now have no control.

Surveillance of CJD was reinstituted in the United Kingdom in 1990 to evaluate any changes in the pattern of the disease that might be attributable to BSE. The overall incidence of CJD has risen in the UK in the 1990s, although this is most likely due to improved ascertainment of CJD in the elderly as a result of the reinstitution of surveillance. In 1993, a project for co-ordination of national CJD surveillance programmes was funded by the EC, linking already established or proposed national registers in France, Germany, Italy, Netherlands and the UK. Initial results reported in 1994 and 1995 revealed similar incidence rates of CJD in all participating countries contrasting with the striking variation in the incidence of BSE at that time, with more than 100,000 in the UK and less than ten in each of the other countries. However, if the epidemiology of a human spongiform encephalopathy acquired from the consumption of contaminated beef or through handling contaminated beef or meat and bone meal is similar to Kuru the incubation period may be dose related and could be up to 30 years. Therefore, a dramatic increase in incidence of CJD related to consumption of beef could yet appear.

In March 1996, the UK CJD Surveillance Unit described a distinct variant of CJD in ten people aged under 42 (average age 27 years) with dates of illness since January 1995. This variant has not been previously recognised and is characterised by behavioural change, ataxia, progressive cognitive impairment and a prolonged duration of illness (up to 23 months) compared to classical CJD. In addition, the EEG is not typical of classical CJD and the brain pathology, although showing marked spongiform change and extensive amyloid plaques, is also not typical. The most striking features of these new cases are the extensive plaque formation and a pattern of prion protein immunostaining which is unique and remarkably consistent between cases. No patient had recognised risk factors for CJD such as iatrogenic routes of exposure or mutations on the prion protein gene. Are these new variants a result of increased ascertainment? It is possible but unlikely that cases of fatal neurological disease in young people would go undocumented. A recent review of the UK register of cases of subacute sclerosing panencephalitis (SSPE) at the Communicable Disease Surveillance Centre has provided no evidence that cases of CJD were misdiagnosed as SSPE. After reviewing the data on these variant CJD cases the UK Spongiform Encephalopathy Advisory Committee (SEAC) advised the Government 'that in the absence of any credible alternative, the most likely explanation at present is that these cases are linked to exposure to BSE material before the Specified Bovine Offal (SBO) ban was introduced in 1989'. The SBO ban prohibits the use of those tissues (brain, spinal cord, thymus, tonsils, spleen and intestine) most likely to contain the infective agent of BSE in products for human consumption. Although no association between consumption of beef and this new variant of CJD has been demonstrated, the question as to whether British beef was safe to eat before the SBO ban, and is safe to eat after the ban, has yet to be answered. Evidence supporting the hypothesis that the BSE agent is responsible for the emergence of the new form of CJD in humans has been provided by a recent report describing similar clinical, molecular and neuropathological features in three BSE experimentally infected macaque monkeys. Since the announcement of the ten variant CJD cases in March 1996, six further cases have been identified in 1996. Molecular typing reveals that the new variant CJD is similar to BSE but different from sporadic CJD, supporting the hypothesis that these new cases are associated with the consumption of contaminated beef.

An individual's prion gene (PrP) type is a major factor in determining susceptibility to the BSE agent. The prevalence of homozygosity for methionine or valine at PrP codon 129 has been reported to be increased significantly in people with sporadic CJD. About 50 people have developed CJD after treatment with contaminated growth hormone or gonadotropins, and they show an increased prevalence of methionine or valine homozygosity at PrP codon 129. The entire population of people exposed to BSE may therefore not be at equal risk of developing the disease: a person's PrP genotype might dramatically influence their risk. Some people may not be susceptible and in others their genotype may result in an incubation period so long that they will have died from old age long before developing a spongiform encephalopathy.

If further human cases of this new variant continue to appear, then we could be witnessing the enfolding of the greatest public health catastrophe ever. There are many lessons for the public health community from this present debacle not least of which is 'how did we let it happen?'.

ANTIBIOTIC RESISTANCE AND HOSPITAL ACQUIRED INFECTIONS

The ability to control organisms with pharmaceutical agents is surely one of the greatest modern challenges in infection. Antibiotics have been used since 1933: their success underpinned the optimism associated with the introduction of the National Health Service in 1948: Development of resistance was widely recognised by the 1950s, but disillusionment and public concern is a new challenge for the 1990s. It is now firmly established as an emerging problem, covering not just the limited viral susceptibility to drugs but the evolution of resistance in old bacterial enemies.

Examples of emerging bacterial resistance include *Shigella dystenteriae*: resistance to nalidixic acid which thwarted the control of dysentery in refugee camps in Rwanda, where thousands died. Rising levels of dysentery in the UK and other developed countries has been a less fatal but nevertheless a devastating public health problem in recent decades. *Salmonellae* have also proved adept at evading antibiotic control; *Salmonella typhi*, for example, is now resistant to most cheap antibiotics, presenting a major control problem in poor countries. In the last five years, trimethoprim and ampicillin resistance have been detected and outbreaks of this multiresistant strain have been reported in India, Pakistan and Bahrain. In addition to *S. typhi*, multiple drug resistance has recently been detected in other *Salmonella*. *S. typhimurium* DT104, has chromosomally integrated resistance to ampicillin, chloramphenicol, streptomycin, sulphonamides and tetracyclines. In England and Wales in 1995 over 87% of strains of *S. typhimurium* DT104 from humans were resistant to these five antibiotics with 26.9% and 6.2% of strains having additional resistance to trimethoprim and ciprofloxin respectively. Another significant development has been the emergence of resistance to fluoroquinolone drugs in the poultry associated serotypes *S. hadar* and *S. virchow*. The use of antibiotics for treatment, prophylaxis and as growth promoters in animals has contributed to the emerging resistance in the non-typhoid *Salmonellas*, progressively reducing in options for the treatment of invasive salmonellosis in humans.

Tuberculosis, the 'white plague' of earlier centuries, has re-emerged in multi-resistant form; both community and hospital outbreaks show that we are poorly prepared and equipped for the threat of *Mycobacterium tuberculosis*, *africanum* or *bovis* as well as less virulent strains that can invade those with impaired immunity. *Staphylococcus aureus* has thrived on the widespread use of antibiotics in developed countries, now susceptible to a dwindling number of topical or parenteral agents; epidemic methicillin resistant *S.aureus* is now established throughout our communities, although still the subject of a thousand control policies in our hospitals.

Streptococci have been slower to develop resistance, but with studies showing that up to 25% of nursery-aged children are colonised with penicillin-resistant *Streptococcus pneumoniae*, the era of streptococcal resistance is already upon us. *Enterococci* have emerged as a major problem in intensive care and bacteraemia, through resistance to vancomycin and other parenteral drugs. *Clostridium difficile* is another nosocomial pathogen responsible for increasing numbers of cases of antibiotic-associated colitis, particularly in the elderly. Gram-negative bacilli have long invaded our hospitals with resistant strains: the list includes *Escherichia coli*, *Citrobacter*, *Pseudomonas*, *Proteus*, *Klebsiella* and *Serratia*; the shift towards community care has challenged labels such as 'hospital opportunist organisms', and it is thought provoking to consider that this shift may be accelerating the spread of antimicrobial resistance.

If the causes of antimicrobial resistance are the way we have used and mis-used these drugs, then is the solution to the challenge partly within our power? Public health specialists can contribute in three main areas: first in helping to establish more efficient surveillance and feedback of information; secondly, in policy development on the responsible use of antibiotics and the monitoring and audit of policies and control procedures. Thirdly, we can use our network of central, regional and local public health epidemiologists to investigate clusters, outbreaks and other emergencies. Surveillance is not simply a local or national matter: we now have the technology and political will to liaise across countries on all these issues. Antibiotic resistance has all the criteria for a worthwhile public health challenge: it is no longer alarmist to predict that lethal epidemics will increase this challenge in the coming years.

INFECTION IN PREGNANCY AND INFANCY: THE FORGOTTEN EPIDEMIC?

Forgotten, no, but definitely moved from centre stage is the risk of infection to the unborn and newly born child. Advancing technology has shifted the emphasis to the problems of prematurity, surgery and other treatment of congenital anomalies. While the hazard of infection is acknowledged, such as by Group B beta-haemolytic *Streptococci*, several factors reduce the ability to prevent or control both sporadic cases and outbreaks. These include the absence of reliable, rapid diagnostic tests for many organisms (not least the new problems raised by HIV in pregnancy and neonates); lack of awareness of infection risks and signs; unknown infections; poor post-mortem information; lack of pharmaceutical agents for viral infections or appropriate therapy for rapid onset cases of fulminating septicaemia. All these lacks are relative and there is welcome continuing advance, particularly in treatment. But added to this array of problems is the apathy of impotence: in the wake of the enormous success of antimicrobials, the remaining infections, even those re-emerging in importance may be perceived as unpreventable.

The recently established Confidential Enquiry into Stillbirths and Deaths in Infancy (CESDI) which covers England has published detailed information on the deaths occurring in 1993 and of trends in 1994 (Department of Health 1995/96). Infection was reported to contribute to 42% of all deaths and 34% of those occurring in the neonatal period, and was the main cause in 28% of deaths. In a subgroup of 388 normally formed large birthweight (>2.49 kg) babies, whose death occurred during or associated with the intrapartum period, the main cause of death was infection in 5.4%; infection was a contributory factor in 19%. CESDI includes an audit scoring system of such deaths, so that lessons can be learned about 'suboptimal care': whereas 42% of the deaths were scored as potentially avoidable, those related to infection were less likely to be scored in this way:

In several of these cases there was apparent delay in starting treatment or in anticipating neonatal infection problems. Panels acknowledged the difficulty of identifying infection, which was rarely the subject of a grade for suboptimal care.(Part I, p35).

By far the largest proportion of deaths in the CESDI 1993 data was death during the antepartum period (35% of all deaths). Only a few (73) of these were subjected to confidential enquiry, so whether infection contributed to the majority with unknown cause of death cannot be assessed. However, in many cases, the diagnosis of unknown cause was established by exclusion, for example, after post-mortem investigation for the absence of congenital malformation; the important role of infection is supported by the high proportion of antepartum deaths of known cause where infection was implicated (23%) (Part II, p.38). Diseases of unknown cause are of interest to public health, and those who specialise in infection may speculate that there is a historical precedent for suspecting as yet unrecognised infections. A case control study of antepartum death currently in progress may produce further clues, but the public health challenge remains.

Where infection occurs after birth, the data are in general better and the public concern, in general, greater. The enormous progress made by immunisation has reduced some infections, but left others still either unpreventable or untreatable in some cases; Group B *Neisseria meningitidis* is an example. The availability of vaccine for Group A and Group C strains has in some ways complicated the control initiatives, again hampered by delays in grouping of isolates, absence of isolates in cases given early antibiotic therapy, and antibiotic resistance in the drugs used to attempt to eradicate carriage.

Viral outbreaks, such as with Coxsackie virus Group A and Respiratory Syncytial Virus, are even harder to control. There is a public expectation, possibly shared by public health specialists, that vaccine development will make other measures unnecessary, and further epidemiological investigation unfruitful. But, meanwhile, outbreaks will continue to occur, and the possibility of a pandemic exists.

VACCINE PREVENTABLE DISEASES

The rapid decline in many of the vaccine preventable diseases demonstrates what can be accomplished with effective public health interventions. However, substantial challenges remain. These relate to sustaining vaccination coverage rates, achieving disease eradication and control targets, establishing a reliable global system for the supply of vaccines and supporting ongoing development of new and safer vaccines. Rapid biotechnical developments have led to the introduction of new vaccines in recent years, e.g. hepatitis B and *Haemophilus* influenza type B (Hib) and there are several vaccines in the pipeline including varicella, rotavirus, conjugate and conjugate meningococcal and pneumococcal vaccines. The ability to manipulate DNA in genetic engineering, construction of multi-antigenic peptides, the development of new adjuvants and the development of new delivery systems such as immunostimulating complexes and biodegradable controlled release devices means that more and more effective and safe vaccines may become available. Vaccines against HIV, *Helicobacter*, Hepatitis C, *Chlamydia*, *Gonococcus*, enteric bacteria and malaria are but a few that, if available, could have a great impact on improving the public health.

The introduction of Hib vaccine into the primary immunisation schedule in the UK in 1992, and the addition of a catch up programme for all children up to 48 months of age, resulted in the rapid decline in the incidence of Hib bacteraemia and meningitis. This successful public health intervention demonstrates what can

be achieved with an effective vaccine and a properly managed programme.

Meningococcal disease reamins to be conquered. It is a spectrum
of illness caused by the Gram-negative diplococcus *Neisseria
Meningitidis*. Meningococcal meningitis has a case fatality rate of 5%
or lower, but septicaemia has a case fatality rate of around 25% (up
to 50% in Waterhouse–Friedrichson syndrome). Between 3 and 5%
of survivors are left with permanent neurological sequelae, most
commonly deafness. In the UK, it is more common during the win
ter months which may be related to the possibility that circulating
respiratory viruses increase the susceptibility to disease. The incidence fluctuates from year to year but since the mid-1980s there has
been an upsurge with typical annual rates of between 2.5 and 3.0 per
100,000. The peak incidence of infection is at six months of age
coinciding with the disappearance of maternal antibody.
Approximately 10% of the population carry the organism in the
nasopharynx at any one time. In the past, approximately 70% of
infections in England and Wales were caused by Group B organism
for which there is no effective vaccine available. However, since
1995, the incidence of Group C cases has been increasing with a
high proportion of the cases in the 5–24 age-group. A vaccine exists
against Group C, although it is ineffective in children under the age
of two years, and provides only short-term immunity above this age,
it can be used to control spread in outbreak situations. The management of clusters poses a difficult challenge for public health
physicians who have often to operate under intense media scrutiny.
Guidelines have been published; however, every outbreak must be
assessed separately with control measures aiming to optimise management of cases, limiting secondary spread from index cases and
providing information to the public to reassure the well and to
ensure early presentation to clinicians by the ill.

Before the introduction of *Pertussus* immunisation in the 1950s,
the average annual number of notifications in England and Wales
was over 50, 000 whereas, in 1972, when vaccine acceptance was
over 80% there were only 2069 notifications. However, in 1975, public anxiety about the safety of the vaccine resulted in acceptance
rates falling to 30% and major epidemics with over 100,000 cases followed in 1977/79 and 1981/1983. Confidence in the vaccine returned
and the incidence declined in 1986 and reached an all-time low of
1873 notifications in 1995.

Acellular vaccines are now available which have a much lower
incidence of side-effects than their whole cell counterparts. They

are already licensed in many countries, although not in the UK. When available in the UK, they will have a role as a booster in older children and also for primary immunisation when given in combination with other vaccines. Acellular vaccines are likely to be considerably more expensive than the currently available preparations

The eradication of polio is likely to be achieved within the next 5–10 years and, if the political commitment existed world-wide, the global eradication of measles and the elimination of neonatal tetanus would also be possible. Disease prevention and control are the objectives of the immunisation programmes, and good-quality surveillance in addition to high coverage rates is necessary to ensure this.

Surveillance of adverse events is becoming increasingly important. As more vaccines are added to the routine schedule with the possibility of vaccine interactions, and as disease incidence declines, there will be increasing public and media concern over the risk of an adverse event being greater than acquisition of the disease.

The resurgence of diphtheria in the former Soviet Union and Russian Federation, and the occurrence of outbreaks of measles and pertussus in the US and poliomyelitis in the Netherlands, are other reminders that a disease close to elimination can return to epidemic proportions. Vaccine service should be extended to the currently unreached, often the residents of some developing countries and marginalised communities in developed countries. These diseases do not respect national boundaries and a united international effort is required. A global coverage of 80% is not acceptable as it leaves pockets of unvaccinated people where the infection can flourish. Maintenance of high vaccine coverage in countries where the disease is no longer a problem is essential as importations, from countries where immunisation programmes are not effectively delivered, could continue to occur for many years.

SEXUALLY TRANSMITTED DISEASES

Using unlinked anonymous and other data, it is possible to estimate the total number of prevalent infections (HIV-1 adults alive). It is estimated that 23,300 HIV infected adults were living in the UK at the end of 1994. When compared to other countries in Southern and Northern Europe the UK has a relatively low population prevalence. Transmission through sex between men accounts for a larger proportion of infections in the UK and the rest of Northern Europe, than in Southern Europe. The intense epidemics seen historically among injecting drug users in Edinburgh and Dundee, and more recently in Southern Europe, have not occurred in England and Wales. In England and Wales, the number of cases of HIV infections acquired heterosexually but not associated with time spent in high prevalence countries are still few and the majority of AIDS cases attributed to heterosexual transmission are associated with having lived in or visiting Africa, emphasising the necessity to provide services addressing the needs of African men and women and their families.

World-wide, the highest rates of new HIV transmission are considered to be occurring in South and South East Asia and to a lesser extent in sub-Saharan Africa. These developments have implications for the UK, given the long tradition of travel between these areas and the UK.

The bulk of current HIV-1 transmission is among homosexual and bisexual men and they remain the highest priority for preventive activities. Particular attention should be paid to younger men who have become sexually mature since preventive messages were first developed in the mid-1980s, but new infections continue to be reported in all age-groups. Intravenous drug users (IDU) remain vulnerable and there is continued need for preventive activities such as needle exchange programmes. Survey results indicate that female IDUs and young IDUs of both sexes are more likely to share injecting equipment.

Unlinked anonymous testing identified a high level of HIV-1 infection among heterosexual men and women attending genitourinary medicine (GUM) clinics and the fact that more than half of those infected were unaware of their infection illustrates the important role of GUM clinics in sexual health promotion and underlines the need for the provision of accessible voluntary confidential HIV-1 testing for patients who present with a possible sexually transmitted disease.

Priority should be given to offering HIV-1 testing during antenatal care to all women in higher prevalence areas such as London, and to all women at higher risk and those requesting testing. The added benefits of diagnosing infection during pregnancy are that the risk of transmission of infection from mother to child can be substantially reduced by interventions such as treatment with zidovudine and by avoiding breast feeding.

Chlamydia trachomatis is the most common curable sexually transmitted pathogen in the UK, with over 39,000 cases treated in GUM clinics in England and Wales in 1995, more than three times the number of cases of gonorrhoea reported. Many cases of chlamydial infection are asymptomatic and go unidentified. Despite its high prevalence (2–12%) in women attending general practices, the epidemiology of chlamydial infections has been incompletely studied and screening, diagnosis and treatment remain inconsistent. Up to 30% of untreated or inadequately treated women may develop pelvic inflammatory disease and, of these, one-fifth may become infertile and one-tenth develop an ectopic pregnancy. Reducing the high levels of genital *Chlamydia* infection and sequelae among the general sexually active population must be made a priority. In addition, reducing the high levels of STDs in young persons and among teenage women, in particular, who experience higher incidences of gonorrhoea, *Chlamydia* infections and genital warts than other agegroups must remain high on the agenda.

ENHANCED SURVEILLANCE

Timely recognition of infectious diseases requires early warning systems to detect these diseases so that investigations can be rapidly initiated and control measures introduced before they become major public health problems. National and international public health networks for effective disease surveillance are necessary if emerging and resurgent infectious diseases are to be recognised. Recent developments in electronic communication have been applied to public health surveillance systems and facilitated progress. The Internet has presented the opportunity for rapid global information exchange at low cost.

CONCLUSION

The public health challenge of infectious diseases is partly of our own making: in public health, we have spread our skills across a wide range of medical, social and political ills, in many cases rather thinly. It behoves health professionals to maintain a population perspective when attempting to prevent and reduce morbidity and mortality and, if we are to maximise the health gain from a limited heath care budget, control of infectious diseases must remain a priority. We must improve the public health infrastructure at district, regional, national and international level. In addition, we must avail of the new developments in molecular epidemiology which have facilitated the tracking of pathogens. The lesson seems to be, that no matter how important the other challenges are for public health, infection must remain amongst the highest priorities, possibly right at the top of the list.

ACKNOWLEDGEMENTS

We gratefully acknowledge the contribution of our colleagues Drs Norman Begg, Angus Nicholl and Nicky Connors in the preparation of this chapter.

REFERENCES

Centers for Disease Control and Prevention 1994 Addressing Emerging Infectious Disease Threats: A Prevention Strategy for the United States. Atlanta, Georgia: US Department of Health and Human Services, Public Health Service
Department of Environment and Department of Health 1990 *Cryptosporidium* in Water Supplies, ed Sir J Badenoch. HMSO, London
Department of Health 1996 Unlinked Anonymous HIV Prevalence Monitoring Programme. England and Wales.
Department of Health 1995 Confidential Enquiry into Stillbirths and Deaths in Infancy; Annual Report for 1 January– 31 December 1993. HMSO, London
Institute of Medicine 1992 Emerging Infections: Microbial threats to health in the United States. National Academy Press, Washington DC.
WHO 1992 Global Health Situations and Projections, Estimates 1992. WHO, Geneva.

10. Screening: A challenge to rational thought and action

Muir Gray

INTRODUCTION

The withered arm of Kaiser Wilhelm II has been the subject of much speculation among those whose historical methods include psycho-analysis. The Kaiser's weakness, it has been argued, made him bellicose and made the First World War inevitable. As is often the case, the explanation is more mundane and mercenary, and the main cause of the First World War was economic as Germany sought to develop an empire to match the British Empire (Evans & von Strandmann, 1988). The appointment of Alfred von Tirpitz as Secretary of State for Naval Affairs in 1897 started 'the Great Naval Race', and in 1902 Lord Selborne, the First Lord of the Admiralty, commented: 'if the German fleet becomes superior to ours then the German army can conquer this country'. Tension was high even in 1902, stimulated in part by this awareness of German foreign policy, and in part by other trivial but no less influential events, notably the Kaiser's telegram to the Boers and the publication in 1903 of the *Riddle of the Sands* (Childers, 1903). This book, like *The War of the Worlds*, caught the popular imagination and sold in very large numbers, fuelling the fear of war.

A closer examination of Germany revealed not only an ambitious foreign policy and the development of a great Navy but also a well-established range of health and social services set up by Bismarck in the 1870s under the broad heading of 'Praktisch Christentum'. Bismarck in the newborn Germany promoted physical exercise in schools, mother and child care, nutrition support for children, and a variety of other measures designed to improve the public health and the health of individuals, both men and women. This knowledge, combined with the evidence that the health of many potential recruits to the Boer War was unsatisfactory, led to the setting up in

Britain of a Royal Commission on Physical Degeneration which focused on measures that needed to be taken to improve child health and led to the Education (Provision of Meals) Act of 1906 and another Education Act in 1907 which started the School Medical Service and introduced child health screening. The strength of the arms of Kaiser Wilhelm II had probably no effect at all upon the events that led up to the Great War; fear of Prussia, on the other hand, undoubtedly had a major effect on child health, and later adult health, in Britain by introducing screening in childhood.

THE DEVELOPMENT OF SCREENING IN THE 20TH CENTURY

In the first half of the 20th century, interest in screening grew, reaching its height in the 1960s when a combination of the availability of automated biochemical testing, the perceived success of the tuberculosis control programme based on 'mass radiography', and the general hubris of that confident and bullish decade, led to a massive upsurge of interest in screening. Wiser heads, however, counselled caution and a landmark report from the World Health Organisation (Wilson & Jungner, 1968) listed the criteria that should be used to assess whether or not a screening programme should be introduced (Box 10.1). These criteria have stood the test of time and still form the basis of the methods used to appraise screening for the 21st century, but they now need modification to take into account the pressures of the 1990s.

Anyone making decisions about health care for groups of patients or populations in the 1990s is operating in a different culture than existed in the 1960s. As the need and demand for health care have increased due to population ageing, the development of new technology, and rising patient expectations, pressures have increased on decision-makers. Decisions are based on three main types of factors which are inter-related and which are shown in Fig. 10.1, and as pressure has increased, decision-making has become more open.

APPRAISING THE EVIDENCE ABOUT THE BENEFITS OF SCREENING

The Wilson and Jungner criterion was that there should be an 'accepted' treatment for patients with a recognised disease. The term 'accepted' was clearly understood in the 1960s but would be unacceptable now, and an analogous criterion would now read that there should be a treatment for which there was strong evidence

Box 10.1   Criteria for appraising screening developed in the 1960s

- The condition sought should be an important health problem.
- There should be an accepted treatment for patients with recognised disease.
- Facilities for diagnosis and treatment should be available.
- There should be a recognisable latent or early symptomatic stage.
- There should be a suitable test or examination.
- The test should be accceptable to the population.
- The natural history of the condition, including development from latent to declared disease, should be adequately understood.
- There should be an agreed policy on whom to treat as patients.
- The cost of case-finding (including diagnosis and treatment of patients diagnosed) should be economically balanced in relation to possible expenditure on medical care as a whole.
- Case-finding should be a continuing process and not a 'once and for all' project.

based on good quality research that the treatment did more good than harm. The good quality evidence on which decisions about screening should be based would be evidence based on either a randomised controlled trial or, preferably, a systematic review of ran-

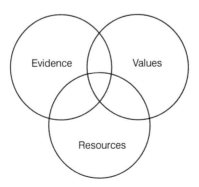

Fig. 10.1   The three decision-drivers.

domised controlled trials, and the reason for the importance of emphasising the need for the randomised controlled trial to be the gold standard research method for assessing the benefits of screening derives from the problem of lead time bias. Fig. 10.2 shows what happens when diagnosis takes place 'earlier' by the introduction of a test that can pick up disease at a presymptomatic stage but which has no impact on the overall duration of the disease; this is called 'lead time bias' and the only way to determine whether or not earlier diagnosis leads to cure and longer survival in a population is to randomise members of that population either to receive the screening programme or not to receive the screening programme.

When assessing the benefit of a programme, it was common to use relative risk reduction in the 1960s but it has been shown that the use of relative risk reduction biases decision-makers. In one elegant study in the United Kingdom, the research workers presented 182 health authority members with results from randomised controlled trials of breast cancer screening and results from a systematic review of cardiac rehabilitation services. They presented the results in four different ways, as shown in Table 10.1. 140 questionnaires were returned and there was clear evidence that the willing-

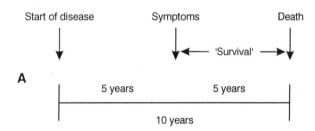

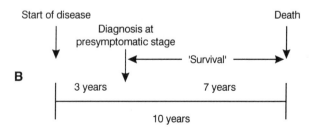

Fig. 10.2 The source of lead time bias.

ness to fund either programme was influenced significantly by the way in which the data were actually presented. Information about relative risk reduction stimulated a significantly higher inclination to purchase, particularly for the screening service where relative risk reduction is high and the absolute benefit is relatively low, as is the case in many screening tests. In presenting evidence in absolute terms, the number needed to treat is an accurate and easily understood measure that is gaining increasingly widespread acceptance.

Table 10.1 Four different ways of presenting the same result to decision-makers

Information presentation	Mammography	Cardiac rehabilitation
Relative risk reduction	34%	20%
Absolute risk reduction	0.06%	3%
Percentage of event-free patients	99.82 vs 99.8%	84 vs 87%
Number needed to treat (NNT)	1592	31

Source: Fahey *et al.*

RESOURCES

The 1960s was an era in which growth in health care spending was, in most developed countries, steady, unremarkable and taken for granted; a different era. In the 1990s, much more attention is paid to costing, particularly to estimating the opportunity costs of a new programme or treatment.

For example, when the National Breast Screening Programme was introduced in the United Kingdom, it was costed accurately, and additional resources were made available to ensure that the programme was set up to provide the adequate level of quality to do more good than harm. Some criticism was, however, made of the Breast Screening Programme on the grounds of opportunity cost with critics arguing that, if the additional resources made available for breast screening had been used to improve breast cancer treatment services, the beneficial effect would have been even greater for the same investment.

As programme budgeting becomes more common in health care, it is probable that this approach will be used more frequently. When, for example, one is assessing the costs of screening for colorectal cancer the type of questions that will be asked, assuming that it was concluded that colorectal cancer screening had a beneficial effect, would be, in the following order.

1. Is there any expenditure on the control of colorectal cancer or its consequences (the 'Colorectal Cancer Control Programme') which is less valuable than the investment of the same amount of resources in colorectal cancer screening?

If the answer is 'yes', the less valuable activity should be stopped to fund the screening; if the answer to question 1 is 'no', a second question should be asked:

2. Before adding additional resources to the budget for the Colorectal Cancer Control Programme to allow the introduction of screening, would the same, or greater, benefit be obtained by adding these resources to some other activity which can prevent colon cancer or improve the diagnosis or treatment of the disease?

If it is considered that additional resources should be added to those already available to control cancer, the decision-maker must answer a third question:

3. From which other part of the general health care budget can we take away resources to add to the Colorectal Cancer Control Programme budget sufficient money to allow screening to be added to the range of interventions without changing the balance of that programme budget?

VALUES

The clinician or public health professional places a high value on the beneficial effects of an intervention. So, too, does the patient or healthy member of the public invited for screening. But, it is increasingly appreciated that patients also place an important value on the adverse effects of health care intervention and they may place a higher value on the adverse effects of health care than do the professionals. This is particularly important in screening where healthy people are invited to participate in a programme which will benefit only a small proportion of them and some of those who will experience adverse effects will not be those who will benefit from the programme.

Furthermore, beneficial effects of screening illustrate the law of diminishing returns, namely for each fixed increase in the number of people covered, or the number of tests per person covered, for example three-yearly testing rather than five-yearly testing for cervical screening, there is a progressively smaller increase in benefit, and the curve relating benefit to resources invested flattens out, as shown in Fig. 10.3.

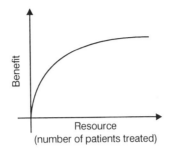

Fig. 10.3   The relationship between screening intensity and benefit.

However, the adverse effects of screening have a linear relation-ship with the resources invested, as shown in Fig. 10.4.

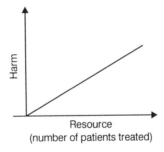

Fig. 10.4   The relationship between screening intensity and benefit.

Thus, as the amount of resources invested increases, the differ-ence between benefit and harm changes, and there may come a point where the adverse effects outweigh the benefits (Fig. 10.5). It is sometimes argued that screening is justifiable even though there

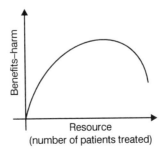

Fig. 10.5   The net effect of screening as intensity increases.

is little evidence of benefit because of the reassurance that is given and because it is felt in some societies that, if there is a probability of benefit, then it is justifiable to introduce a screening programme. In general, attitudes towards screening are more positive in the United States than in the United Kingdom and the decision to introduce a screening programme is made at a lower threshold.

CRITERIA FOR THE 1990s

Taking into account all these factors, it is possible to add to the criteria introduced in the 1960s and listed in Box 10.2 are additional

Box 10.2   1990s criteria for appraising screening

Is there evidence from a good-quality RCT, analysed on an intention-to-treat basis, that the proposed screening programme is effective in reducing mortality?
If the answer is 'no', there is 'no' case for implementation.
If 'yes', the following questions should be addressed.

- How many people have to be screened to find one case or prevent one death (the number needed to treat: NNT)?
- How many people would be adversely affected by screening:
        per thousand screened;
        per life saved?
- How broad are the confidence intervals around the estimated size of the beneficial effect, and what are, at each end of the confidence intervals, the:
NNT;
numbers adversely affected?
(This question is particularly important because the size of the effect found in the ideal circumstances of the trial may not be reproducible in a routine screening service.)
- What are the financial costs of the screening programme, and what health benefits would be obtained by using those resources allocated to screening on:

(a) other ways of managing the health problem the
        screening programme has been designed to tackle,
        for example, improving the treatment of breast cancer;
(b) other services for that population the screening pro-
        gramme is designed to benefit;
(c) any other service for any other population group?

criteria that can be used for appraising screening in the 1990s.

Decisions about screening policy are now made much more care-fully with explicit justification for these decisions which are, to a degree, culture-specific with the result that each country needs to interpret the evidence and take into account their own values and the resources available. For this reason it is probably necessary for there to be similar reports from, for example, the USA (US Preventive Services Task Force, 1996) and Canada (Health Canada, 1994).

However, in all countries the evaluation is becoming more rig-orous with greater emphasis on cost-effectiveness, taking into account both the opportunity costs and the full costs of screening (Russell, 1994; Haddix et al., 1996). The full costs of screening include the costs of false-positive test results on the health and well-being of those people who have positive results but who do not have the disease for which the screening test was designed (Quilliam, 1992).

MANAGING FOR QUALITY IMPROVEMENT

Having made the decision that a screening test should be intro-duced, the public health professional has to ensure that their popu-lation receives screening of an adequate quality to do more good than harm. Research evidence is often provided from high-quality, highly motivated screening programmes and this is not necessarily reproducible in practice. If quality is low, adverse effects may be higher and beneficial effects lower. This changes the shape of the curves described in the previous section and, more importantly, changes the relationship between them, and with low quality screening it may be that the adverse effects outweigh the benefits (Fig. 10.6).

There is, however, reassuring evidence that the benefits pro-duced by research workers can be reproduced in practice (Hakama et al., 1997).

For these reasons it is vitally important for any screening pro-gramme to be managed so that it achieves adequate levels of qual-ity and for the public health service either to manage the programme directly, based on the principles of total quality man-agement, or for them to ensure that any screening offered their population is subject to external quality assurance schemes and achieves results that are above the standard required to do more good than harm.

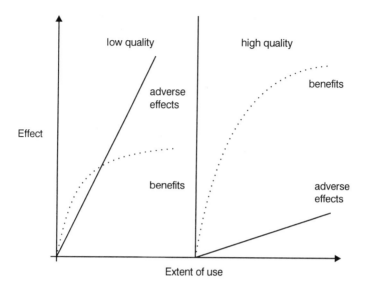

Fig. 10.6   Benefits and risks of low and high quality screening. (Source: Moore *et al.*, 1994.)

MANAGING SCREENING PROGRAMMES

Much prominence has been given to screening tests but, from the public health perspective, it is essential to think only of the screening programmes – all those steps, from the identification of the relevant population to the final diagnosis and treatment, which have to be co-ordinated to do more good than harm.

To do this, it is essential to set up systems to ensure that the population is offered only programmes that are able to do more good than harm, and that the programmes are delivered at levels of quality which ensure that the theoretical benefit demonstrated in research studies is reproduced in the ordinary service setting.

Systems have to be set up to allow potential programmes to be identified and for their introduction to be controlled so that only those programmes for which there is good evidence that they can do more good than harm are considered for introduction, and so that they are not actually introduced until sufficient resources have been identified, for example, trained personnel, to ensure that theoretical benefit is achieved. In every country there are, of course, screening programmes in place for which there are not good quality assurance systems, namely systems which do not have explicit quality criteria, information systems to allow the level of performance of screening programmes to be measured and compared with the standards, and managerial authority to allow action to be taken if a screening programme falls below the acceptable standard.

As resources get tighter and public expectations rise, it will be essential for public health services to manage screening policy and quality more explicitly and openly.

REFERENCES

Childers E 1903 The Riddle of the Sands. Reprinted 1993 as a Wordsworth Classic, Ware, Herts
Evans RJW, von Strandmann HP 1988 The Coming of the First World War. Oxford University Press
Fahey T, Griffiths S, Peters RJ 1995 Evidence-based purchasing. British Medical Journal 311: 1056–60
Haddix AC, Teutsch SM, Shaffer PA, Dunet DO 1996 Prevention Effectiveness. A Guide to Decision Analysis and Economic Evaluation. Oxford University Press
Hakkama M, Pukkala E, Keikkila M, Kallio M 1997 Effectiveness of the Public Health Policy for breast cancer screening in Finland. British Medical Journal 314: 839–912
Moore A, McQuay H, Muir Gray JA (eds) 1994 Testing a screening test. Bandolier 1(5): 1–6
Quilliam S 1992 Positive Smear. 2nd Edn, Charles Letts & Co
Russell LB 1994 Educational Guesses. Making Policy about Medical Screening Tests. University of California Press
The Canadian Task Force on the Periodic Health Examination 1994. Clinical Preventive Health Care. Canada Communication Group Publishing
US Preventive Services Task Force 1996 Guide to Clinical Preventive Services. 2nd Edn, Williams & Wilkins
Wilson JMQ, Jungner G 1968 Principles and Practice of Screening for Disease. World Health Organisation, Geneva

11. Developments in Mental Health

Hilary Guite, Graham Thornicroft, Kay Beaumont

INTRODUCTION

Mental health policy has developed so rapidly and intensively over the last decade (see Table 11.1) that it can be a difficult area to break into for public health specialists. Fortunately, there are now three key texts Conway *et al.*, 1994, Thornicroft & Strathdee 1996 and Kings Fund, 1997 which, supplemented by the Cochrane database of mental health reviews, together provide a comprehensive overview.

The first part of this chapter aims to provide a brief summary of the main developments in general adult mental health practice in the health services over the last decade. The second part of the chapter focuses on the main issues for public health specialists who work in the mental health field.

MENTAL HEALTH DEVELOPMENTS

Deinstitutionalisation

Care in the community of people with severe mental illness is often portrayed as a failure by the media. However, in the mental health field, care in the community has involved two different processes, one a relative success, the other a relative failure. Closure of mental hospitals has resulted in the resettlement in the community of large numbers of mainly older adults who had been institutionalised. This has been a relatively well-planned and resourced programme. In contrast, the development of an infrastructure of services to care for the new long-term sick, who are mainly younger adults, has been haphazard and poorly resourced.

Given the current pressure for re-opening mental institutions, it is worth briefly recapping the reasons for their closure. The case for the closure programme arose from a combination of developments in understanding of mental illness, the development of anti-

Table 11.1   Mental health policy and funding developments 1986–1996

1986	Making a reality of community care. Audit Commission	Identified the lack of transfer of resources from hospitals to community.
1988	Report of the committee of inquiry into the care and aftercare of Miss Sharon Campbell. Spokes J.	First of the series of public homicide inquiries. Recommended improved interagency working and development of guidelines for good practice for discharge and aftercare.
1990	Caring for people. Community care in the next decade and beyond HMSO. London. White paper NHS and Community Care Act 1990	Framework for local authority lead for community care from 1993. Care management introduced which includes: assessment of need, the purchase and co-ordination of services. Local authorities directed to spend 85% of money transferred to them from the DSS budget on the independent sector.
1991	Care Programme Approach. HC (90) 23 LASSL (90)11	Guidelines for systematic arrangements for the assessment and aftercare of people referred to specialist psychiatric services, involving a systematic assessment of health and social care needs, a care plan (with user involvement), an identified key worker, and regular review.
1991	Mental Illness Specific Grant	Payment to local authorities (who make a 30% contribution) to increase the level of social care available to people with severe mental illness.
1991	Defeat depression campaign	RCGP sponsored national campaign offering information and training opportunities on the management of depression in primary care.
1992	Mental Illness Key area in 'Health of the 'Nation'. HMSO	Targets set for reductions in suicide in the general population, in people with severe mental illness and for improvements in the health and social functioning of mentally ill people.
1992	Review of services for mentally disordered offenders. Reed J. DH/HO. HMSO	Mentally disordered offenders should receive care and treatment from health and social services rather than custodial care. Led to the development of court and prison diversion schemes.
1993	Secretary of State's 10-point plan for developing safe and successsful community care	The plan included a review of legal powers, development of standards in the care of schizophrenia and commissioning of mental health services (produced in 1995 by the Clinical Standards Advisory Group), new training for key workers and the introduction of the supervision registers.
1994	Mental health nursing review. Butterworth	Identified the central importance of the service user in the planning and monitoring of mental health services.

Table 11.1 *continued*

1994	Finding a place. Audit Commission	Critical report which identified poor targeting of services on those in most need.
1994	Introduction of supervision registers for mentally ill people. HSG (94) 5	Development of a local register of patients at risk of serious self neglect, suicide or serious harm to others.
1994	The report of the inquiry into the care and treatment of Christopher Clunis. Ritchie JH *et al.* HMSO	The most influential of the homicide inquiries which identified similar problems to those found in the Sharon Campbell inquiry in 1988.
1994	Guidance on discharge of mentally disordered people and their continuing care in the community. HSG 94(27)	Placed particular emphasis on risk assessment. Required health authorities to set up an independent inquiry in all cases of homicide by a patient known to specialist psychiatric services.
1995	Building Bridges (DH) HON	Principles and guidelines to the practice of inter-agency working
1996	Patients in the community. (Mental Health Act). Supervised discharge.	New powers of supervision in the community, similar to guardianship but includes the power to convey.
1996	Mental health challenge fund	£10 million central funding for new evidence-based service developments which is matched £ for £ by health authorities.
1996	Spectrum of care, 24-hour nursed beds, audit pack for CPA. HSG (96)6, LASSL (96) 6	A summary of key elements of comprehensive local mental health services, guidance to purchasers and providers about increasing provision of 24-hour nursed beds and an audit pack for the CPA
1996	HoNOS: Health of the Nation Outcome Scales. Wing JK *et al.* RCP Research Unit. 1996	Final version of the HoNOS which has good psychometric properties. 12-item scale which measures four areas: behavioural problems, impairment, symptomatic problems, social problems

psychotic medication and finally a series of inquiries in the 1970s and early 1980s which identified the problems facing these large institutions (Martin, 1984) (see Box 11.1).

The outcomes of the closure programme for individual patients has been comprehensively monitored in North East London by the TAPS (Team for the Assessment of Psychiatric Services) (Dayson, 1994; Leff, 1994). Positive findings on long-term follow-up show that the majority of patients prefer their new homes, and on average patients are increasing their social networks by one new friend each year. A review of adverse outcomes showed that less than 5% had any contact with the police. Importantly over 95% were followed up and none of these was homeless. (Dayson, 1994; Leff, 1994).

Box 11.1   Problems with the large mental hospitals identified by inquiries in the 1970s and 1980s

---

Systematic ill-treatment of patients by some members of staff, which included assaults on patients;
Theft from patients and the hospital;
Isolation from scrutiny and lack of internal complaints procedures;
Patients deprived of contact with friends and relatives;
The corruption of care from the primary aim of treatment to secondary aims of the preservation of order, quiet and cleanliness;
Lack of respect for patient individuality, little involvement of patients in planning their treatment;
Failures of professional leadership;
Failures of administration and general management;
Staff shortages;
Defensive practices by unions;
Poor training.

Source: Summarised from 'Hospitals in Trouble'. J.P. Martin.

In the UK there has been a steady reduction of over 120,000 mental health beds since 1960 (Davidge et al., 1993). However, the hospitals did not begin to close until the 1980s. The majority have planned closure dates in the 1990s. The closure of the hospitals has removed a safety valve for fluctuations in acute admissions and has led to a 'concentration effect' (Patrick et al., 1989) of people with psychosis on acute admission wards making the wards more difficult to manage. This has made it difficult to release staff into community settings.

Development of Community Mental Health Teams

With the development of locally based psychiatric services on District General Hospital sites, psychiatric services were able to define geographical catchment areas for which they provided services. Mental health sectors cover populations of 50,000 people on average (up to double this in areas of low need). In most districts these sectors are served by Community Mental Health Teams (CMHTs). There was little strategic input into the development of these teams and the role and function of them vary greatly, depending on local circumstances. The teams consist usually of psychiatrists, community mental health nurses, psychologists, occupational therapists, support workers and often social workers. Many teams had open access policies and developed good links with primary care teams often providing services on a sessional basis in selected practices. A number of problems have arisen with these teams:

- there has been 'role drift' towards the care of people with less severe mental illness with subsequent little or no impact of the teams on needs for in-patient care;
- there is no or little co-ordination with in-patient care;
- few CMHTs have developed case registers of the most severely mentally ill with primary care practices despite close links;
- the allocation of sessions to primary care is poorly correlated with need;
- few teams have managed to fully integrate care planning under the Care Programme Approach and Care management carried out by social workers;
- over-reliance on unfocused counselling and support by CPNs with no formal training in counselling;
- reduction in family work by social workers because of the demands of their assessment role under care management[1]
- low levels of provision of effective treatments such as compliance therapy (Kemp, 1996) and psychosocial interventions (Lam, 1991) and cognitive–behavioural therapies (Effective Health Care Bulletin, 1993);

The four main responsibilities of CMHTs should be :

- the assessment of new referrals, including referrals for needs assessments and for assessments under the Mental Health Act 1983 for compulsory admission;
- the provision of on-going support and effective health and social interventions to people with severe mental illness (this should ideally be 7 days a week);
- the provision of focused effective psychological therapies;
- the provision of a crisis response (including managing access to crisis accommodation).

---

[1] In 1993, social services departments were given a statutory duty under the NHS and Community Care Act to assess the needs of people for social support to live in community settings. The care received can attract charges and can be provided by local authority, voluntary agencies or private companies. The purchase and co-ordination of this care is known as care management.

In addition, the CMHTs carry out, with in-patient teams, the needs assessment, care planning and review required for local authority care management and the Care Programme Approach. If CMHTs also have control over hospital beds, length of stay is reduced.

The Care Programme Approach and the Supervision Register

The Care Programme Approach (CPA) introduced in 1991 (see Table 11.1) provides a pragmatic structure to reduce the chance of patients with mental illness losing contact with services and to ensure that the full range of their health and social needs are addressed. It also seeks to ensure that patients and their carers are involved with the development of care plans, know who to contact and that they receive co-ordinated care. Implementation of the CPA initially increases length of stay as unmet needs are identified. Subsequent experience shows that this declines and that the numbers of people remaining in contact with services significantly increases. A key benefit is a reduction in homelessness as a result of rent arrears (personal communication David Roy, 1997).

Other benefits are likely to accrue as more attention is paid to the nature of the care provided (see next section) by teams and key workers.

Since April 1994, patients who are thought by the consultant psychiatrist to be particularly at risk of self-harm, self-neglect or harm to others are supposed to be entered on to a supervision register. Identification of these risk factors is difficult and open to considerable variation in interpretation. No new resources followed the introduction of supervision registers, the registers are not shared routinely with other agencies or districts and therefore many psychiatrists have found it difficult to understand what benefits the supervision registers may have in addition to a well-functioning CPA and CPA register. There are very large variations between districts in the numbers of people entered onto the supervision register depending on the interpretation of psychiatrists of the purpose of the register and local guidelines for entry and exit from the register. The supervision register is currently being evaluated by a team at the Institute of Psychiatry to determine how it is being implemented at a local level and to provide recommendations for improving the system. The study is due to report by the end of 1997.

Effective Interventions in the Care of People with Severe Mental Illness and Core Components of a Comprehensive Service.

Conway, Shepherd and Melzer reviewed the evidence of effectiveness of interventions in mental illness in 1994 and 1996. They emphasise the synergistic nature of interventions in the care of people with severe mental illness and the importance of the context within which services are provided for the efficacy of treatments in non-trial situations. Box 11.2 gives a list of interventions which have been proven to be effective in randomised controlled trials in the treatment of people with severe mental illness. This list reflects the interests of those currently most active in research and therefore misses many nursing, social work and other professional interventions which may be effective but have not yet been evaluated. Box 11.3 lists components of care considered to be core to the provision of mental health services for people with severe mental illness in addition to the interventions tested by randomised controlled trial. A later section of this chapter covers some innovative approaches to care and treatment led by the voluntary sector and user movement.

Mentally Disordered Offenders and Others Requiring Similar Services

Mentally disordered offenders and those requiring similar services are people with a mental disorder who have been arrested or who have behaviours which could lead to arrest. The publication of the Reed report in 1991, which clearly stated that the majority of mentally disordered offenders should be cared for by general adult psychiatric teams, stimulated transfers from prisons to hospitals of mentally disordered offenders within a year of publication (Table 11.2). There are three common misconceptions about this group of patients:

- mentally disordered people offend and present through the criminal justice system as a result of too early discharge to 'community care';
- the problems faced by the health services in providing services for mentally disordered offenders are the result of the prison service 'offloading' a group of prisoners who are really their responsibility;
- the increasing numbers are a result of over enthusiastic psychiatric staff who are conned by people who would rather be in hospital than in prison.

Box 11.2. Interventions in mental health care of people with severe mental illness which have proven effectiveness from randomised controlled trials

---

Organisation of care
Assertive community outreach; [a]
Day hospital care;
Case management in the long term; [b]
Initial assessment at home or in a community setting by two people from different disciplines.

Therapeutic interventions
Antipsychotic drugs;
Clozapine for patients who are resistant to classic antipsychotic therapy;
Lithium for acute mania (but long-term outcome is not necessarily improved by prophylactic lithium therapy);
Continuous low dose depot medication with additional oral doses at times of stress
Compliance therapy; [c]
Psychosocial interventions — packages of care which include educational, behavioural and cognitive elements with the client and their family to reduce expectations, improve problem solving and improve communication;
Effective for families both with and without high EE (expressed emotion); [d]
Social skills training (assertiveness, conversational skills, problem solving, medication management) as part of a long-term programme of support.

Source: Conway, Shepherd & Melzer (1996).

---

[a] Frequent outreach, copious practical and social support, training in daily living skills, appropriate medication, 24-hour crisis intervention, access to temporary emergency housing and respite beds.
[b] Case management is a mechanism for ensuring continuity of care and co-ordination of service provision for those with long-term care needs and in effective studies has included practical support and a therapeutic relationship. Effectiveness is limited by the quantity and quality of services available to the client.
[c] Education about drug treatment for schizophrenia, combined with cognitive therapy to identify erroneous beliefs and unhelpful patterns of thought and challenge these with competing explanations and behaviour therapy to alter maladaptive ways of coping (Kemp et al., 1996).
[d] Expressed emotion — highly emotionally involved and critical communication.

Box 11.3   Other core components of mental health services for people with severe mental illness.

Housing with adequate support, ranging from 24-hour staffed residence to mainstream local authority or private housing with support;
In-patient beds;
Welfare benefits and financial advice;
Physical and dental care;
Behavioural–cognitive therapy for psychotic symptoms (small studies so far look promising);
Rehabilitation;
Practical skills and support;
Work and education or other meaningful daytime occupation;
Ordinary social contact in recognised social roles, e.g. with local shops and facilities and neighbours;
Support for carers.

Source: Adapted from Strathdee & Thornicroft (1996).

In contrast to the myth, Table 11.2 shows that there were more mentally disordered offenders transferred from prisons in 1974, at a time when few beds had closed and lengths of stay were long. The numbers of people transferred from prisons fell not as a result of bed closures but as a result of the movement towards unlocked wards. This left fewer suitable places for transfer of patients who were potentially violent or likely to abscond. The problem of insufficient secure accommodation was identified as early as 1974 by the Glancy report (Department of Health and Social Security, 1974) which recommended that 1000 new medium secure beds be opened[2] and the Butler report (Home Office and Department of Social Security, 1975) which revised this figure to 2000 places. By 1992 even the Glancy target had not been met.

The psychiatric literature in the 1980s carried reports of the sometimes intolerable conditions that patients with severe mental illness were kept in while waiting transfer to a suitable NHS place (Kings Fund, 1997). Furthermore, some patients were detained in

[2] Medium secure beds are beds where security is provided by higher staffing levels than acute wards, by security policies and by a locked and secure environment.

Table 11.2 Number of people with mental disorder transferred from prison to psychiatric hospitals between 1974 and 1994

Year	1974	1985	91/92	92/93	93/94	94/95
Number transferred to psychiatric hospital	1209	546	390	648	774	715

Source: Bowden (1990) and HM Prison Service (1996). Copied from London's mental health. King's Fund with permission.

prison simply for a psychiatric assessment only to be rejected by the services. Finally, the majority of mentally disordered offenders transferred from prison are known to the psychiatric services before their arrest. Between two thirds and three quarters have had a previous psychiatric admission and a diagnosis of a psychotic disorder.

The Reed report advised that schemes be set up to divert people with mental illness from four main points in the criminal justice system:

- at first contact with the police;
- in custody;
- in court;
- in prison.

Much progress has been made in setting up court diversion schemes but provision of psychiatric services within prisons is more patchy (Kings Fund, 1997).

People requiring medium secure care can be costly to Health Authorities — the average cost per person per year in the South Thames Region in 1996 was £95,000. Rates of use of medium secure beds vary 20-fold within districts in London (Guite & Field, 1997). Variations in unemployment alone explain 49% of the variation between districts. The problem is particularly acute in districts with large African and Caribbean populations as well as high unemployment since these groups are over-represented within medium secure services.

Homicide Inquiries and Assessment of the Risk of Violence

The first widely available public inquiry into a homicide by someone with a mental illness was published in 1988. The inquiry was about the killing of a psychiatric social worker at Bexley hospital in London by Sharon Campbell, a young woman with a psychotic disorder. The recommendations included improvements in care planning, joint working between agencies and across other administrative boundaries, key worker allocation, multi-disciplinary review, better risk assessment training, training in the management of people from different ethnic backgrounds and the development of a register of patients who are vulnerable and require special supervision. In 1994 Health Authorities were instructed to set up an inquiry into any homicide by people who had been in contact with specialist psychiatric services. Between 1992 and 1996 there have been 26 published inquiries which have reiterated similar recommendations to those made in the inquiry into the care of Sharon Campbell. Nearly half of these inquiries have been in London. Each of these inquiries has cost the Health Authority around £250,000 and, in conjunction with more explicit guidance about consultants' responsibilities for risk assessment, has led to changes in admission and discharge thresholds (Roy *et al.*, 1996).

The responsibility for all dangerous behaviour by patients is gradually being forced on to health, social services and probation services, yet there is no evidence that they can predict violence in general psychiatric populations or reduce the chances of violence. All inquiries call for better risk assessment for violence. The problem facing clinical staff is that the sensitivity of risk factors for the prediction of violence is about 80%. This means that, even with the best systems, 20% of violence is not foreseeable. These risk factors for violence are also common in non-violent groups of patients. The specificity is only about 30% meaning that at least one in three people identified as potentially violent will not be so. In acute psychiatric populations, the prevalence of serious violence is low and risk prediction becomes worse than chance. There is no specific intervention to reduce risk of violence. Admission into crowded wards puts other patients and staff at risk. The best hope for reducing risk of violence is better recording of details about previous violence and improvements in the general care planning and the management of specific risk factors for individuals. This requires increased communication between professions and agencies and probably more resources unless prior violence is to become a means to gain access to care.

Social Services

Many of the above changes and developments in mental health have affected social services jointly with health services. However, there have been two major changes in social services this decade: the development of the ASW (approved social worker) role and the introduction of needs assessment and care planning for community care.

In the previous decade following the Seebohm report (1968) psychiatric social workers were removed from employment by hospitals to employment by local authorities in generic social services departments. Recognition that mental health social work was receiving a lower priority than child-care work within these generic teams and that social workers needed more training to be able to carry out their role with respect to involuntary hospital admissions led to the development of the requirement for social workers to be approved to have 'appropriate competence in dealing with people who are suffering from mental disorder'. Approved social workers (ASWs) receive a minimum of 60 days of training. Their role is defined in the Mental Health Act 1983 (MHA) and further refined in the Codes of Practice and by case law (which is regularly reviewed by Jones, 1997).

The importance of the independent role of the ASW is that, under the law, they are required to consider 'all the circumstances of the case, including past history of the patient's mental disorder, his present condition and the social, familial and personal factors bearing on it, the wishes of the patient and his relatives and medical opinion'. They must also ensure that a full range of options have been considered before committing someone to hospital. Under the MHA 1983 local authorities must appoint sufficient numbers of ASWs to carry out the functions given to them by the Act.

The 1990 NHS and Community Care Act gave local authorities the responsibility for assessing needs for care in a community setting and for co-ordinating this care but not necessarily providing it. This is known as the brokerage model of care management. Not requiring social service departments to provide care has stimulated a greater range of providers including voluntary, not-for-profit and commercial providers in the mental health field. Under Community Care legislation, anyone is eligible for a needs assessment and for a care plan, but many local authorities publish eligibility criteria in order to manage demand. Carers of people with severe mental illness have a right to an assessment of their own needs under the Act. Local authorities can charge for services and the amount can vary between boroughs.

The additional responsibilities for needs assessment and care management for social workers has meant that access to social services for general advice is more difficult now than a decade ago. Other agencies such as citizens' advice bureaux and benefit agencies and, in some cases, solicitors have taken on this advice role. Other changes in practice have been a reduction in family work and general social contact with clients previously provided by social workers.

Housing

Changes to housing legislation — in particular, the shift of responsibility for social housing from local authorities to housing associations — has led to an overall increase in rents. Reduced availability of low cost rented accommodation and stricter criteria for access and maintenance of tenancies, which many housing associations require, has meant that people with severe mental illness find it difficult to obtain a tenancy or keep one they have. Local authorities have fewer properties as a result of the 'right to buy' scheme and the development of a mixed economy of provision of social housing. During the 1980s and early 1990s local authorities did not significantly increase the provision of special needs housing placements for people with mental illness (Government Statistical Service, 1993). Hostel accommodation can be counterproductive and/or unacceptable to people with severe mental illness, further reducing options for many people. People assessed under care management not to require supported accommodation may also not be eligible or thought capable of maintaining a local authority or housing association tenancy. Joint working between housing, social services departments and health services can help to overcome some of these problems by arranging appropriate support, review and access to help in a crisis.

Voluntary Sector and User Movement

The voluntary sector has become a major provider of services, particularly housing, residential advocacy and day support services. Carers report that access to voluntary sector self-help groups for relatives, information leaflets and telephone support lines are most useful (LSL, 1997).

The user movement in mental health has become increasingly organised, vocal and effective. Box 11.4 summarises the views of users about the service system they need (Beeforth & Wood, 1996).

The new charter for users of mental health services for implementation in 1997 begins to address some of these issues, but Beeforth and Wood advise the development of a local charter which covers a statement of intent, confidentiality about information, safety (including safety of medication by avoiding over prescription), complaints

Box 11.4   Ten priorities for services from a user perspective.

Access to information;
Presence of a charter;
24-hour, 7-day a week availability;
Practical help;
Flexibility and responsiveness to individual need;
User run services;
Advocacy;
Access to specialist help;
Something meaningful to do during the day;
An integrated system with continuity of care.

Source: Beeforth & Wood (1996).

procedure, needs-led service — availability of options and involvement in decision-making and the type of service received, and support to achieve a desirable standard of quality of life.

User-led services are beginning to define new approaches to service delivery. These attempt to provide services which are responsive to users' needs such as social and economic recognition and control over their treatment. Some examples are given below.

Shanti

This is a service aimed particularly at the needs of black women. The work of the project has encompassed broader issues such as the social, economic and political context of mental health and marginalisation of groups of people. Results of an evaluation showed that the service was catering mainly for people with depression but also a sizeable proportion have psychotic symptoms. At a minimum of 2 years after treatment, 75% of women had maintained symptom reduction (Shanti, 1993).

Clubhouse

This is a model where users provide day-time occupation, hold fully paid jobs between groups of patients and provide support and advice.

Hearing Voices Groups

These are groups which help users manage their auditory hallucinations through cognitive processes.

Client-centred groupwork

Psychologists taking a client-centred approach to group work with women who have been sexually abused in childhood have shown that women who have not found mainstream services helpful have made significant progress using focused group work (Watson *et al.*, 1996).

The user and voluntary movement provide many different approaches to residential provision. Most of these emphasise the importance of individual needs as the basis for the service.

Mental Health in Primary Care

The maximum time spent in formal training about mental health for over half of all UK general practitioners is 8 to 12 weeks as a medical student. Whether a hospital based post-registration job in psychiatry (just under half of new principals) helps general practitioners manage primary care mental health problems is not known, but there is no doubt that most GPs are poorly prepared for managing the 15% to 25% of their case load who present primarily with a mental health problem (Fry, 1985; Strathdee & Jenkins, 1996). Mental health issues have been judged to be important in consultations for other reasons, and studies have shown that about half of patients with clinical depression are missed in general practice. The 'role drift' of community mental health teams (p.173) towards care of the less severely mentally ill and the slow development of practice-based registers of people with severe mental illness is therefore not surprising, given the scale of the mental health problems in primary care and the relative lack of training to deal with it.

In addition to an increase in staff from specialist mental health services working in general practice, there have been four other main developments in primary care mental health in the last decade:

- changes in prescribing — a decrease in use of benzodiazepines (e.g. valium) and an increase in the use of specific serotonin reuptake inhibitors (SSRIs) (e.g. Prozac);
- an increase in practice-based counsellors;
- fund holders purchase of mental health services;
- educational programmes and mental health facilitators.

Changes in prescribing

Benzodiazepine hypnotics and minor tranquillisers replaced barbiturates for the treatment of anxiety and insomnia in the 1970s. Use of benzodiazepines reached a peak in 1979 when there were 30 million prescriptions for benzodiazepines (Smith & Jacobsen, 1988). Realisation that long-term use impairs memory and affects driving skills (five-fold increase in road traffic accidents), and that there was a benzodiazepine withdrawal syndrome has led to some reduction in prescribing (Smith & Jacobsen, 1988).

Prescriptions for specific serotonin reuptake inhibitors (SSRIs) such as fluoxetine 'Prozac' have increased in the 1990s. They are as effective as tricyclic antidepressants for the treatment of mild to moderate depression and have the advantage of causing less drowsiness (*Prescribers Journal*, 1996). Their major advantage is that they are safer in overdose. The disadvantages are that they are not as effective for the treatment of severe depression, which is known to be underdiagnosed in primary care and SSRIs cost about ten times as much as tricyclic antidepressants.

Increase in practice-based counsellors

By 1992, up to one-third of all practices provided access to counselling (Winkler & Burnett, 1996), but provision bears no relation to need (Kerwick *et al.*, 1997). Counselling in primary care is thought not to be effective (Effective Health Care, 1993). There is some evidence that part of the reason for the poor effectiveness are the low levels of formal training in those providing counselling (Fallowfield, 1993). This includes Community Psychiatric Nurses who do not routinely receive practical training in effective counselling techniques. There is clear evidence that non-focused counselling is ineffective, but there is good evidence that targeted counselling, e.g. for bereavement or relationship problems, brief problem-solving techniques and cognitive behavioural therapy are effective (Effectiveness Bulletin, 1993).

Fund holders purchase of mental health services

GP fund holders can purchase out-patient treatment and referrals to all members of mental health teams (excluding local authority social workers). Ford and Sathyamoorthy's study of fundholding in 1996 showed that this resulted in an increase in referrals of people with less severe mental illness to CMHTs and fewer referrals of patients with psychosis for whose services GPs had to pay. Many fund holders have arranged for consultant psychiatrists to provide outpatient sessions within the practice, but Strathdee and Jenkins (1996) have shown that, on average, each consultant psychiatrist serves the needs of 15 GPs and if all requested a similar service would preclude psychiatrists from actively managing people with severe mental illness. GP fund holding of mental health services has further increased the inequity of access to mental health services.

Educational programmes and mental health facilitators

The joint 'Defeat Depression Campaign' between the Royal College of General Practitioners and the Royal College of Psychiatrists in 1991 aimed to improve the recognition of depression in primary care and the use of symptom checklists to guide diagnosis and management. Antidepressant prescribing has increased since then. There is still a vigorous debate about the most appropriate dose of antidepressants, uncertainty about when to commence treatment and which patient groups are most likely to benefit and widespread belief that antidepressants are addictive (Paykel & Priest, 1992; Kendrick, 1996; BMJ Letters, 1997). In one study of increased identification of depression, no patient benefits were found (Dowrick & Buchan, 1995).

Mental health facilitators in primary care have been shown to be effective in increasing knowledge of external support, developing a programme of educational activities, development of practice protocols, and increasing recognition of mental illness (Kerwick *et al.*, 1997). Most primary care mental health facilitators have a nursing background, but the RCGP has set up a number of national mental health fellowships to attract doctors into this area. The new RCGP unit for mental health education in primary care based at the Institute of Psychiatry has set up a training course for GP continuing medical education tutors and their nearest nurse facilitator/trainer.

Mental Health Commissioning

Most mental health commissioning is carried out by health authorities, although the increased budgets of joint commissioning groups has encouraged more joint planning with social services.

A review of mental health commissioning by the Health Advisory Service showed that only a third (35%) of health authorities in England and Wales in 1993/4 and 1994/5 had a mental health strategy (Cumella *et al.*, 1997). Lack of knowledge within their purchasers was seen as a problem by the majority of NHS trusts, though not by purchasers themselves.

Multi-agency working

In 1995, the Department of Health produced guidance about inter-agency working for people with severe mental illness called 'Building Bridges' (Department of Health, 1995). This describes the principles on which joint working should be based: a shared definition of severe mental illness, a commitment to multi-agency training, senior management commitment and a commitment to joint commissioning wherever possible, a focus on the needs of service users and carers, a joint strategy, well-understood access to health and social services, a system for regular interchange of information between agencies and regular review of joint agency working. Building Bridges supports joint working on the Care Programme Approach, the supervision register, and shared information systems.

A recent Green Paper 'Developing partnerships in mental health' (DH, 1997) aims to address some of the structural problems to shared commissioning. Four options are proposed:

- the mental health and social care authority. The creation of a new authority.
- single authority responsibility. Either health or local authority given responsibility for commissioning.
- a joint health and social care body. A new body which remains accountable to the local authority for funds allocated for social care and to the health authority and GP fund holders for funds allocated for health care.
- agreed delegation. Health and local authorities agree to delegate particular functions or responsibilities to each other. Accountability arrangements remain as at present.

The Green Paper options all relate to adults with severe mental illness. Given the problems of defining the severely mentally ill and that people move between categories, this could cause problems in practice. The Green Paper does not address the interface with housing departments and housing associations nor other voluntary groups.

MENTAL HEALTH ISSUES FOR PUBLIC HEALTH SPECIALISTS

The developments in mental health policy and understanding of mental health services over the last decade define many of the main issues which public health specialists should be dealing with in adult mental health services. These include:

- poor targeting of mental health services geographically, between severe and less severe mental illness and between ethnic groups;
- low levels of implementation of effective service models and treatments;
- the need to develop the capacity in primary care to effectively manage less severe mental illness and to share in the management of people with severe mental illness;
- the requirement to develop services for mentally disordered offenders;
- the need to develop and implement a jointly developed comprehensive strategy for mental health services in partnership with service users and providers, social services and housing departments and voluntary groups;
- the resource implications of requirements by fund holders and non-fund holders for practice based care for people with less severe mental illness;
- the Health of the Nation targets, monitoring of strategy implementation and outcome monitoring and a broader approach to mental health promotion including the impact of environment, employment and deprivation on mental health;
- low levels of confidence in commissioners by mental health providers.

However, the work of many public health specialists is dominated by approval of extra-contractual referrals for acute and secure beds, needs assessments for specialist services and contracting meetings since these cause the greatest pressure on health authority managers. With the increasing development of a primary care-led NHS, it will be interesting to see what role is retained for public health specialists in mental health and what scope there will be for developing the public health agenda of equity, effectiveness and health promotion.

The following section concentrates on two issues which are likely to remain important topics for public health specialists: needs assessment and, in particular, prediction of needs for in-patient beds and the mental health Health of the Nation targets including outcome measurement.

Epidemiological Needs Assessment

There are now a comprehensive set of sources (see following sections) from which to estimate local prevalence of mental health problems and take into account how needs vary with different levels of socio-economic deprivation. Estimates of local prevalence should be based wherever possible on sources which account for variations in socio-demographic factors rather than national norms. Local data should be used to supplement estimates, particularly in areas of high and low social deprivation where predictions are less stable.

Severe mental illness and bed numbers

Mental illness needs index (MINI)

This is a computer program (available on disc from the Royal College of Psychiatrists research unit), which provides an estimate of the number of people likely to be admitted to mental hospital at least once each year. It works by calculating the extent of socio-demographic factors which have been shown to predict admissions in each local ward and by combining these to compute the MINI index and the predicted numbers of people admitted at least once within a year. The MINI index can be useful for identifying similar districts locally and assessing the rank of need for the district and the rank of need for sectors within a district. The numbers of people admitted can be useful to compare against the current numbers of people admitted each year. The MINI is a better predictor of need for mental health admissions than the Jarman score.

The MINI has been used to predict bed numbers and other components of mental health services by applying the index to a range of suggested norms for components of mental health services. Two sets of norms are used, based on a review of the literature and on the judgement of experts and are dependent on the current state of implementation of the service developments listed in Box 11.2 at the time of the publication or expert view. Most of the effective components of care listed in Box 11.2 reduce requirement for inpatient beds. The effectiveness of the interventions in Box 11.2 is synergistic and therefore it is difficult to predict their precise impact on needs for inpatient beds at any one point in time. Many of the interventions reduce requirements for in-patient beds by reducing the length of admission as well as by reducing the need for admission. Revised ranges for norms of current in-patient beds have been included in the MINI following the work of the King's Fund commission on London's mental health services when it was found that the index under-predicted need in inner city areas where lengths of stay were short but prevalence of severe mental illness much higher than predicted. These are available from PRISM at the Institute of Psychiatry. As service developments are funded, the need for beds is likely to change.

Length of stay is as important as prevalence in determining the number of beds required within a district. For example, a district with an average length of stay twice that of comparable districts could either admit twice as many patients to the same beds or reduce beds by half by reducing length of stay to the average. The factors which predict length of stay are different from those which predict prevalence of mental disorder. They include clinical practice relating to admission, discharge and care planning, the presence of bed management policies and designated bed managers, the accessibility of social care assessments and the availability of mainstream housing tenancies as well as supported residential care.

Local information

There is therefore no reliable guide to prediction of bed numbers and commissioners need to combine information from the MINI predictions of people admitted with the information about the use of existing beds. The Contract Minimum Data Set and other information specified under contracts can usually be used to find out:

- the length of stay of acute admissions and the number staying over 6 months;
- the number of readmissions within 1 month and 3 months of discharge and the average length of stay of readmissions;
- the proportion of admissions with a primary diagnosis of psychosis;

Other useful information includes CPN caseloads and attendance at day hospitals and day centres.

A local One Day Census of Beds, such as that carried out by the Thames Regions in 1994 (Fulop, 1995) can be useful in providing a profile of bed use including:

- the level of supervision required by current in-patients;
- the percentage who have received a social services assessment;
- the percentage with a care plan.

This information combined with a prediction of prevalence, local knowledge of the extent of implementation of innovations listed in Box 11.2, local development and use of bed management strategies and availability of residential care and tenancies will help estimates of likely future needs for in-patient beds. Needs for in-patient beds tend to increase following public inquiries into homicides as this process can undermine normal clinical decision making at admission and discharge (Roy *et al.*, 1996). Other factors which are important for planning local provision are the needs of different ethnic groups, who may find the development of separate services a pragmatic way of ensuring their needs are met.

Sector level needs assessment

The Care Programme Approach register may provide some information about the number of people with complex needs, but definitions vary between districts and between consultants as there are no standard definitions for entry and exit to different levels of the register. However for planning resource allocation at sub-district level it provides a useful starting point for case identification of people with severe mental illness. Combined with information from general practitioners and residential nursing homes and hostels for people with mental illness it should be possible to identify individuals in need of complex and long term care. The numbers of adults involved are manageable and amount to around 500 per 100,000 adult population (up to half this in areas of low socio-economic deprivation) (Conway *et al.*, 1994).

Less Severe Mental Illness and Primary Care Access to Specialist Mental Health Services

Allocation of CPN time and availability of counsellors in primary care are not related to population size or any measure of need (King's Fund). In the past, health authorities have estimated needs for mental health care in general practice, based on data from the GP morbidity surveys (RCGP, 1995). This provides aggregate national rates. Since the publication of the first report of the OPCS Surveys of Psychiatric Morbidity In Great Britain in 1995, it has been clear that prevalence of less severe mental illness is higher in deprived areas as is prevalence of severe mental illness, though the actual predictive factors differ. The Department of Health has commissioned further work to assess the feasibility of deriving a model to predict prevalence of significant mental health symptoms and clinical depression at the level of postcodes. Early findings suggest that about half the variation in prevalence between postcode areas can be predicted by census variables. If this work can be completed, it will be an enormous help to public health specialists whose only other sources of data of need in primary care are dependent on recognition of the mental illness by the GP and on appropriate treatment and referral. These other sources of data are prescribing data, data about referral to specialist mental health services and a few practices who collect practice based morbidity data using Read coding.

Health of the Nation Mental Illness Targets and Other Outcome Measures

Two of the 1992 Health of the Nation mental illness targets relate to suicide.

1. To reduce the overall suicide rate from 11.00/100,000 by at least 15% by the year 2000.
   Data defined by the Health Service Indicators (HSI) are collected about this target and published in the Public Health Common data set and the Health of the Nation. As well as deaths from suicides, age-standardised rates are given which, in addition to suicide and self-inflicted injury, include deaths from injury undetermined whether accidentally or purposely inflicted since identification of deaths from undetermined causes varies between coroners.
2. To reduce the overall suicide rate of severely mentally ill people by at least 33% by the year 2000.
   The National Confidential Inquiry into Suicides and Homicides has been organised on a national level by the University of Manchester since 1995. It aims to identify all suicides and undetermined deaths within a district and to find how many of these suicides have ever had contact with specialist mental health services. Where there has been contact, professional staff are sent a confidential inquiry form to identify risk factors and service contact prior to the death. It is not clear how severe mental illness

will be defined or identified within districts in order to assess the suicide rate of the severely mentally ill, but such comprehensive identification of the suicide rate of those in contact with services will provide useful data for assessing the relationship between mental health services and suicides.

The final Health of the Nation target is proving more difficult to measure.

3. To improve significantly the health and social functioning of mentally ill people.

The Health of the Nation Outcome Scale (HONOS) (see Table 1, 1996) has been produced and shows good psychometric properties in field trials. It is not known how useful the data will be over longer time periods, whether it will be useful for inter-district comparisons since no data are collected about case-mix and whether aggregate results of outcomes for different services and patient groups will provide useful information for monitoring service improvements.

It may be that, to gather good-quality data on service outcomes, people need to be employed specifically to collect it and the outcomes should relate to specific service groups and include more comprehensive measures of patients' quality of life and their satisfaction with services.

Future developments

In the last decade there have been enormous changes in understanding mental health services, the management of mental health problems and in mental health policy. Need for mental health services can be predicted in a way not possible even a decade ago and there is good consensus about the components of effective mental health services for people with severe mental illness. The danger is that the appropriate increased priority to people with severe mental illness comes as a result of reductions in access to effective treatments for people with less severe mental illness rather than as a result of reductions in ineffective or inefficient treatment. There is no consensus about the components of a service and the appropriateness of care under the NHS for people with less severe mental illness. Ensuring equity of access to effective treatment for people both with severe and less severe mental health problems should be an important public health task and there is a major role for an alliance of people working in mental health in different agencies to advocate for this.

One area which has been neglected partly because of lack of evidence about effective interventions has been primary mental health promotion, i.e. the prevention of mental ill health, although the relationship between socio-economic deprivation and mental ill health is consistent and not solely due to drift following the onset of mental illness. The development of greater awareness by key decision-makers of the importance of the social, financial and physical environment on mental health should be a first step to increasing demands for research into innovative interventions to reduce the prevalence of mental health problems.

REFERENCES

Beeforth M, Wood H 1996 Purchasing from a user perspective. In Commissioning Mental Health Services. eds. G Thornicroft, G Strathdee HMSO, London
Bowden P 1990 Mentally disordered offenders. In Principles and Practice of Forensic Psychiatry. eds. R. Bluglass & P. Bowden. Churchill Livingstone, Edinburgh
BMJ Letters 1997 Eleven letters published in response to Kendrick's BMJ leader. British Medical Journal 314: 826–9
Conway M, Melzer D, Shepherd G, Troop P A 1994 A companion to purchasing adult mental health services. Anglia and Oxford Regional Health Authority
Conway M, Shepherd G, Melzer D 1996 Effectiveness of interventions for mental illness and implications for commissioning. In Commissioning Mental Health Services. eds. G Thornicroft, G Strathdee HMSO, London
Cumella S, Williams R, Sang B 1997 How mental health services are commissioned. The NHS Health Advisory Service survey of commissioning. In Commissioning Mental Health Services. ed. G Thornicroft, G Strathdee HMSO, London
Davidge M, Elias S, Jayes B, Wood K, Yates J 1993. Survey of English Mental Illness Hospitals. 1993 Prepared for the mental health task force. Interauthority comparisons and consultancy University of Birmingham.
Dayson D 1994 Long stay patients discharged to the community — followed up at 1 year, 2 years and 5 years. TAPS (Team for the Assessment of Psychiatric services) 1994, 9th annual conference. TAPS, London
DHSS 1974 Report on Security in NHS Hospitals (The Glancy report) HMSO, London
Department of Health and Home Office 1991 Review of Health and Social Services for Mentally Disordered Offenders and Others requiring similar services. (The 'Reed Report'). The reports of the Service Advisory Groups, an Overview. Department of Health, London
Department of Health 1995 Health of the Nation. Building Bridges
Department of Health 1997 Developing Partnerships in Mental Health. The Stationery Office. CM 3555.
Dowrick C, Buchan I 1995 Twelve month outcome of depression in general practice: does detection or disclosure make a difference? British Medical Journal 311: 1274–6
Effective Health Care Number 5. 1993 The treatment of depression in primary care. University of Leeds
Fallowfield L J 1993 Evaluation of counselling in the National Health Service. Journal of the Royal Society of Medicine 86: 429–30

Ford R, Sathaymoorthy G 1996 Team Games. Health Service Journal 27th June 32–33. Quoted by Kerwick *et al.*, 1997

Fry J 1985 Common Diseases. Their Nature, Incidence and Care. 4th Edn. MTP Press, UK

Fulop N 1994 Psychiatric bed census. South Thames Region Kensington, Chelsea and Westminster Public Health Department, London

Government Statistical Service 1993 Residential support for people with mental illness and people with learning disabilities. Local authority supported residents. Year ending 31 March 1993.

Guite H F, Field V 1997 Mentally Disordered Offenders. Chapter in King's Fund London's Mental Health. The report to the King's Fund London Commission. Johnson S, Ramsay R, Thornicroft G, Brooks L, Lelliott P, Peck E, Smith H, Chisholm D, Audini B, Knapp M, Goldberg D

HM Prison Service 1996 Prison Health: Report from the Director of Health Care

Home Office DHSS 1975 Interim report of the committee on abnormal offenders (The Butler report) HMSO, London

Jones R 1997 Mental Health Act Manual. Sweet and Maxwell London 5th edn

Kendrick T 1996 Prescribing antidepressants in general practice. British Medical Journal 313: 829–30

Kemp R, Hayward P, Applewhaite G, Everitt B, David A. 1996 Compliance therapy in psychotic patients: randomised controlled trial. British Medical Journal 312: 345–9

Kerwick S, Tylee A, Goldberg D 1997 Mental health services in primary care in London. Chapter in King's Fund 1997. London's Mental Health. The report to the King's Fund London Commission. Johnson S, Ramsay R, Thornicroft G, Brooks L, Lelliott P, Peck E, Smith H, Chisholm D, Audini B, Knapp M, Goldberg D

King's Fund 1997 London's Mental Health. The report to the King's Fund London Commission. Johnson S, Ramsay R, Thornicroft G, Brooks L, Lelliott P, Peck E, Smith H, Chisholm D, Audini B, Knapp M, Goldberg D

Lam DH. 1991 Psychosocial family intervention: a review of empirical studies. Psychosocial Medicine 21: 423–41

LSL 1997 Towards a primary care NHS. Lambeth, Southwark and Lewisham Health Authority

Leff J 1994 One year in the community — report on the outcomes of a whole hospital long stay population. (TAPS) 1994 9th annual conference. London TAPS

Martin J P 1984 Hospitals in Trouble. Blackwell, Oxford

Meltzer H, Gill B, Petticrew M, Hinds K 1995 The prevalence of psychiatric morbidity among adults living in private household. OPCS Surveys of Psychiatric Morbidity in Great Britain. Report 1. HMSO

Patrick M, Higgit A, Holloway F, Silverman M. 1989 Changes in an inner London psychiatric in-patient service following bed losses: a follow up of the East Lambeth 1986 survey. Health Trends 21: 121–3

Paykel E S, Priest R G 1992 Recognition and management of depression in general practice: consensus statement. British Medical Journal 305: 1198–1202

Prescribers Journal 1996. Symposium: prescribing for the psychiatric patient in the non-specialist setting. Volume 36, number 4. The Stationary Office, London.

RCGP/OPCS/DH Morbidity statistics from general practice: fourth national morbidity study, 1991–1992. HMSO, London

Roy D, Elliot P, Guite H 1996 Inner City Mental Health. NHS Trust Federation

Seebohm report 1968 committee on local authority and allied personal social services. HMSO, Great Britain

Shanti 1993 Evaluating Shanti. A women's community psychotherapy service. King's Fund and West Lambeth Health Authority, London

Smith A, Jacobsen B (eds) 1988 The Nations Health. A strategy for the 1990s. A report from an independent multidisciplinary committee. Health Education

Authority, London School of Hygiene and Tropical Medicine and King
Edward's Fund for London

Strathdee G, Jenkins R (1996). Purchasing mental health care for primary care. In
Commissioning Mental Health Services. eds. G Thornicroft, G Strathdee
HMSO, London

Strathdee G, Thornicroft G 1996 Core components of a comprehensive mental
health service. Chapter in Commissioning mental health services. HMSO,
London

Thornicroft G, Strathdee G (eds) 1996 Commissioning Mental Health Services.
HMSO, London

Watson G, Scott C, Ragalsky S J1996 Refusing to be marginalised. Group work in
mental health services for women survivors of childhood sexual abuse.
Community and Applied Social Psychology 6: 385.1–14

Winkler F, Burnett A 1996 General practice and the purchasing of mental health
services. In Commissioning Mental Health Services. eds. G Thornicroft, G
Strathdee HMSO, London

12. The Effectiveness Revolution and Public Health

Andrew Stevens and Ruairidh Milne

INTRODUCTION

If the focus of a discipline can be judged by its language, public health has undergone a recent revolution. The terms systematic review, meta-analysis, health technology assessment, clinical practice guidelines, health gain, cost-effectiveness, evidence-based medicine, evidence-based health care, and indeed evidence-based anything, were seldom if ever used in public health practice before the 1990s. And, a host of other terms encompassed by the effectiveness revolution — randomised controlled trials (RCTs), quality adjusted life years (QALYs) and priority-setting — were in relatively limited specialist use in preceding decades.

There is a proliferation of new journals dealing solely with the evidence base of health care (*ACP Journal Club, Cochrane Library, Evidence-based Medicine, International Journal of Technology Assessment in Health Care, Bandolier*, and others). Conferences on the subject are being arranged at an unprecedented pace (notably, the annual Cochrane Colloquia, the biennial Scientific Basis of Health Services and the annual meeting of the International Society of Technology Assessment in Health Care). Even more important, there is serious investment in strengthening the evidence base of health care, both in the UK (with, for example, the UK Cochrane Centre, the NHS Centre for Reviews and Dissemination, the National Co-ordinating Centre for Health Technology Assessment) and abroad (for example, the US Congress Office of Technology Assessment [1], the Agency for Health Care Policy and Research and the Swedish Council on Technology Assessment in Health Care (SBU).

Collectively, these ideas and activities are beginning to amount to a sea change in the thinking around health care (Evidence Based

---

[1] Although discontinued in 1996, its activity survives in other dispersed US units

Medicine Working Group, 1992). This new thinking has started to have an influence on those engaged in clinical academic research and on those delivering health services. In particular, it has struck a chord with those who have population health responsibilities and who straddle both research and service delivery: those involved in public health. We call the new thinking 'the effectiveness revolution' and the aim of this chapter is to consider its meaning, its origins and its implications for public health practice. The effectiveness revolution embraces a wide new terminology, but three critical terms are *cost-effectiveness analysis*, *evidence-based medicine* and *health technology assessment*. They overlap considerably but they stem from different traditions and are therefore worth exploring further.

Cost-effectiveness analysis

This term (also cost minimisation, cost-utility and cost–benefit analysis[2]), derives from health economics, the central theme of which is the scarcity of resources and the need to make choices (Mooney, 1986). Every investment in health care has an 'opportunity cost': that is, the benefit which would have been gained from the resource's best alternatives (Drummond, 1993). The measurement of both costs and benefits is therefore central to health economic research. Health economics has grown rapidly from the mid-1970s to the present. The recognition well beyond health economics, and especially in public health, of cost-pressures has greatly widened the appeal and influence of the contribution of health economics.

Evidence-based medicine

This has spawned the wider term evidence-based health care, but has its roots in the clinical setting as a way of defining and resolving clinical problems. It has been defined as 'the conscientious, explicit and judicious use of current best evidence in making decisions about the care of individual patients. The practice of evidence-based medicine means integrating individual clinical expertise with the best available external clinical evidence from sys-

---

[2] Cost-minimisation (where costs only are measured) is used to compare different costs for equally effective interventions for the same client group. Cost-effectiveness (where outcomes are measured in disease specific units) is used for comparisons of interventions for the same patient group. Cost-utility (where outcomes are measured in generic units) allows any health interventions in principle to be compared. Cost-benefit gives outcomes monetary values and allows comparisons beyond health care.

tematic research' (Sackett *et al.*, 1996). Its intellectual origins go back to 19th century Paris, although it has its recent roots in clinical epidemiology, and particularly in Cochrane's critique of effectiveness and efficiency (Cochrane, 1972). This has been boosted by other suggestions that effectiveness should not be taken for granted, particularly from the growing literature on unexplained geographical variations in clinical practice especially of elective surgery such as hysterectomy and tonsillectomy (Wennberg, *et al.*, 1987). There is also important evidence of a long time-lag between proof of a treatment's benefit in clinical trials and recognition of this in textbooks or other reviews (Antman *et al.*, 1992) (see Table 12.1). The common feature of these ideas is a concern with clinical effectiveness rather than with cost-pressure, but it is only a short step from such clinical concerns to a policy concern with both.

Table 12.1 Evidence on the impact on mortality of thrombolytic therapy (e.g. streptokinase) after myocardial infarction

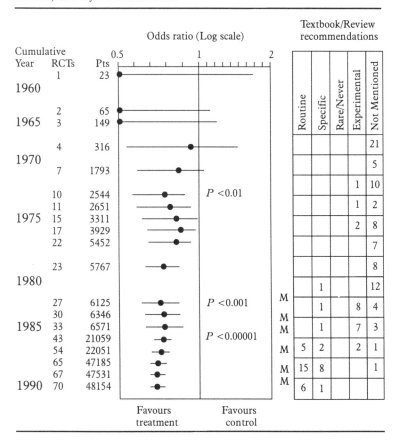

Note to Table 12.1
The use of thrombolytic therapy for people with myocardial infarction, except where there are important contraindications, is now encouraged by experts and routine practice in UK hospitals. A ground-breaking paper published in 1992 by Antman and colleagues (Antman *et al.*, 1992) showed, however, how slowly it was that the results generated by high quality research were incorporated into 'conventional expert wisdom': a necessary precondition for wide uptake in practice.

Antman and colleagues used two complementary methods. First, they identified 'conventional expert wisdom' by looking at review articles and textbook chapters and seeing what recommendations these made about the use of thrombolytic therapy in acute myocardial infarction. These recommendations are summarised on the right-hand side of Table 12.1. It was not until 1986 that a majority of experts recommended the use of thrombolytic therapy. Secondly, they identified all the randomised controlled trials they could find of the use of thrombolytic therapy in acute myocardial infarction and produced a cumulative meta-analysis of the results. With the benefit of hindsight, they were able to show that the benefits of thrombolytic therapy in reducing mortality could have been clear in 1975, more than a decade before experts were recommending this treatment.

Their stated conclusion was modest: 'Discrepancies were detected between the meta-analytic patterns of effectiveness in the randomized trials and the recommendations of reviewers'. More starkly, we believe that they highlighted the dreadful mistakes that traditional reviews, relying on expertise and not a systematic review of the evidence, can make. It seems possible that many thousands of people with myocardial infarction died in the 1970s and 1980s who would have lived if the evidence about the benefits about thrombolytic therapy had been reviewed more systematically.

Health Technology Assessment

This is the term used internationally in which the focus is the production of evidence with both a clinical and policy relevance. Its origin was in the United States, where the Office of Technology Assessment was set up in 1972 to report to Congress on the potential effects — both beneficial and harmful — of (in the case of health care) medical interventions (US Congress Office of Technology Assessment, 1994). Health technology assessment programmes now exist not only in the USA, but also in many European countries including Britain (Department of Health, 1996). They are limited in some to producing systematic reviews of existing evidence with policy implications, but in others (including Britain) they extend to funding, where appropriate, primary research, particularly randomised controlled trials. In all, they draw heavily on pre-existing and increasingly stretched health services research resources which include epidemiologists (both clinical and population), health economists, statisticians, public health practitioners and social scientists.

These three traditions (the academic concern with cost-effectiveness, the clinical concern with evidence of effectiveness and the policy-driven health technology assessment) have a common goal. The goal is cost-effective health care that produces net benefit to patients at a cost that is acceptable to the individual and to society. This goal is approached through a continual interplay between practice and research, as shown in Fig. 12.1. The use of valid and relevant research findings to inform practice is the province of evidence-based health care, while ensuring that research is driven by the needs of policy and practice encompasses both health technology assessment and cost-effectiveness analysis.

THE EFFECTIVENESS REVOLUTION AND PUBLIC HEALTH

Three Possible Reasons for the Association Between Effectiveness and Public Health

The first is the *mission* of public health, such as that espoused in the Acheson report (Committee of Enquiry into the Future of the Public Health Function, 1988), which describes public health as 'the science and art of preventing disease, prolonging life and promoting health through the organised efforts of society'. Such a mission would be impossible without a focus on what is effective and what is not. Furthermore, if it is accepted that the resources available to society are bounded, the population focus of public health necessitates thinking about alternative ways of distributing the same resources. In short, notions of cost-effectiveness are never far removed from the delivery of effective public health.

Secondly, the *location* of public health practitioners has always associated them with health care planning. Indeed, in Britain, the recent NHS changes have explicitly established many of them in commissioning settings, where both costs, through contract pressures, and effectiveness, through the identification of health care

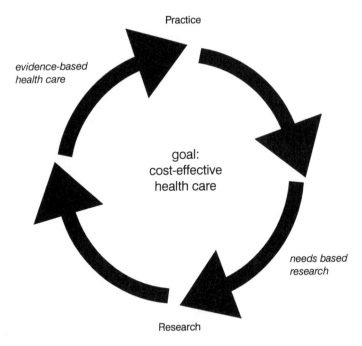

Fig. 12.1 Evidence-based health care and needs-based research.

needs, are day-to-day concerns.

Thirdly, the *skills* of public health practitioners are often accurately targeted at the evidence-based agenda. Such skills cover not just epidemiology and statistics but also increasingly include proficiency with the currency of health (case-mix and outcomes), elements of health economics and of health service research, and a wide clinical knowledge. All of these are being voraciously consumed both by the health technology assessment movement, and by local health care purchasers.

It may also be that evidence-based health care has an intrinsic interest to many public health practitioners. As an approach, it allows public health practitioners a way of going beyond the necessity of balancing costs and spending to the higher goal of striving for the greatest health gain for the population. And, the complex issues of establishing the evidence base and finding ways of bringing it to practitioners and policy makers, has great appeal as an academic activity.

Recent History

When looking at the roots of public health's interest in issues of effectiveness, two things are clear. First, this interest antedates current talk of both evidence-based medicine (Evidence Based Medicine Working Group, 1992) and evidence-based purchasing (Milne & Hicks, 1996). Secondly, it is based on a sound understanding of the importance to good public health practice of knowing both about the health problems of a population and about the cost-effectiveness of services available to help those problems. This is, of course, parallel to the need for clinicians to have access to good clinical information and to up-to-date medical knowledge (Wyatt, 1991).

Early classics

The early classics adopted into the public health literature were, if anything, more concerned with the limits of effectiveness in health care than the practice of public health has been until recently. Illich's 'Limits to Medicine' (Illich, 1976) and McKeown's 'Role of Medicine' (McKeown, 1979) both urged restraint in ascribing effectiveness to unevaluated medical interventions. Cochrane (1972) translated such concern into an agenda for action with his 'Effectiveness and Efficiency: Random reflections on the health service' (Cochrane, 1972). His advocacy of the randomised controlled trial, which acknowledged too, its principal limitations, was a turning point for medicine, which often till then barely justified the label 'science'.

Acheson report

These powerful arguments were, for many years, not acted on by the majority of public health practitioners. One reason for this may have been that, although public health practitioners are concerned with the health of groups and populations, there existed for the first 40 years of the National Health Service no formal population focus at the level at which key planning decisions were taken. This changed with the publication in 1988 of the report Public Health in England ('the Acheson report') (Committee of Enquiry into the Future of the Public Health Function, 1988) which included the novel but crucial sections:

Briefly, the public health responsibilities of district health authorities can be summarised as follows:

To review regularly the health of the population for which they are responsible and to identify problems. To define objectives and set targets to deal with the problems in the light of national and regional guidelines.

As well as the population focus, the Acheson report talked about outcomes:

The central tasks of the DPH [Director of Public Health] and his/her colleagues are as follows:
To provide epidemiological advice to the DGM [District General Manager] and the DHA [District Health Authority] on the setting of priorities, planning of services and evaluation of outcomes

Working for patients

The Acheson report had great significance for the specialty of public health medicine and helped it to prepare for the much bigger changes ('the NHS reforms') heralded with the White Paper *Working for Patients* published in 1989 (Secretaries of State for Health, Northern Ireland and Scotland, 1989). In view of the centrality of the 'purchaser–provider' split to the evolution of these changes, it is remarkable that purchasing was not identified as one of the White Paper's seven key measures. Instead, it was mentioned almost as an afterthought, tucked away in a small paragraph as a by-product of the development of self-governing (Trust) hospitals:

DHAs can then concentrate on ensuring that the health needs of the population for which they are responsible are met; that there are effective services for the prevention and control of diseases and the promotion of health; that their population has access to a comprehensive range of high quality, value for money services; and on setting targets for and monitoring the performance of those management units for which they continue to have responsibility. (section 2.11)

Needs assessment

Working for Patients was not a blueprint; instead, it set in train a period of organisational upheaval in the National Health Service that is only now showing signs of abating (Ham, 1996). That it had so little to say about purchasing mattered surprisingly little. Instead, what 'purchasing' might mean in a publicly funded health service was worked through by health authorities and fundholders across the country, supported by a project team within the Department of Health (DHA Project, 1991). From early on, it was clear that two characteristics distinguished purchasing from previous planning functions in the NHS: the responsibility for the health of a defined population; and the ability to take a detached view of the value of the services offered by health care providers.

Of particular interest to public health was the notion in *Working for Patients* of needs assessment. 'Needs' in health care has a long history (Stevens & Gabbay, 1991) but there was a risk early on in the NHS changes that district public health practitioners would see 'needs assessment' chiefly in terms of measuring morbidity. Pragmatically, the Department of Health project team urged DHAs to assess needs in terms of a population's ability to benefit from health care, and therefore to consider both the incidence and prevalence of health problems and the cost-effectiveness of services available to help those problems (DHA Project, 1991). This approach, which argues that cost-effectiveness should take precedence whenever it is in doubt, has been taken forward in the health care needs assessment reviews commissioned by the Department of Health and targeted at all those concerned with assessing and meeting health care needs (Stevens and Raftery, 1994, 1997).

With the new needs assessment and the effectiveness revolution sharing the theme that effectiveness is frequently in doubt in clinical practice, many public health practitioners have over the last few years taken up an interest in effectiveness. A recent review of the impact of the NHS reforms (written from outside public health) comments: 'it is likely that the current emphasis upon the purchase of clinically effective services derives, at least in part, from the new culture generated by the public health involvement in the purchasing function' (Robinson, 1996). The involvement of public health practitioners in many of the main initiatives associated with the effectiveness revolution, in the UK at least, confirms that view (see pp.215–221).

KEY FEATURES OF THE ASSESSMENT OF EFFECTIVENESS

The effectiveness revolution is not just a matter of marshalling people's energy and enthusiasm towards ensuring effectiveness in health care. It is also about generating the evidence for effectiveness in a worthwhile way. There are three groups of features that contribute to this, each of which has a close association between public health and the effectiveness revolution: those that concern the *relevance* of the evidence; hose that concern the *validity* of the evidence; and those that concern the *delivery* of the evidence.

Relevance is related to the *mission* of public health. Both the population perspective and the emphasis not only on prolonging life but also on preventing disease and promoting health make the case for:

- a broad view of what aspects of health care are to be assessed;
- targeting research resources for maximum population benefit;
- assessing effectiveness in terms of patient relevant outcomes; and
- also measuring the cost so that opportunity costs are borne in mind.

Ensuring the validity of the evidence portfolio both draws upon and adds to public health *skills*. Validity is ensured by:

- the explicit grading of the evidence;
- the systematic review of the evidence; which includes
- the critical appraisal of the evidence; and
- methods for integrating different pieces of evidence.

The delivery of the evidence falls frequently to public health, at least in part because of public health practitioners' *location* close to the commissioning of health services where they are the main professionals with both a service and an academic perspective. Knowledge of the effectiveness of health care needs to be:

- interpreted and delivered appropriately.

Each of these characteristics is elaborated below. While none of them is exclusively in the public health domain, collectively they put public health close to the centre of the effectiveness revolution.

Broad View

The effectiveness revolution in general, and the term 'health technology assessment' in particular, take a broad view, both of health care (including disease prevention and health promotion, diagnosis, acute care, long-term care and rehabilitation) and of health care 'technologies' (covering not just drugs and devices, but all types of intervention including procedures and settings in health care) (Department of Health, 1996; US Congress Office of Technology Assessment, 1994). Nor is the term confined to specific interventions such as surgical procedures. It is also used to mean area-wide and diffuse interventions, such as management systems, information technology and even arguably variants of health care organisation such as the purchaser–provider split.

Targeting

The scope for health care evaluation, like health care itself, far exceeds the resources currently available. The initiative, therefore, needs to be targeted at the most important topics with the biggest holes in the evidence base. In the UK Health Technology Assessment programme, for example, targeting of research resources is achieved by a careful identification and prioritisation effort aimed at filling the NHS's most prominent knowledge gaps. The prioritisation criteria include the burden of disease (both morbidity and cost) as well as the absence of existing evidence (Department of Health, 1996).

Patient Relevant Outcomes

An essential feature of the revolution is its focus on outcome measures relevant to patients rather than intermediate outputs or processes. Research based solely on process and intermediate outcomes has relatively little to contribute to improving the public health unless there is a proven connection between these and patient well-being. For example, the measurement of CD4 counts rather than AIDS symptoms in HIV and the measurement of bone density in osteoporosis rather than fracture rate would have to be carefully justified. In the case of the use of β-interferon in multiple sclerosis (Box 12.1), one of the most optimistically promoted 'outcomes' was of a changed lesion appearance on MRI scans. It is not at all clear how this relates to disease progression. Furthermore, Donabedian's well-established triad of structure, process and outcome (Donabedian, 1973) has been considerably refined in the effectiveness revolution to distinguish different levels of assessment of outcome: efficacy, effectiveness, cost-effectiveness (and cost-utility) as well as overall impact of health care (Box 12.2).

Outcomes can be further elaborated by disaggregating and analysing alternative measures of effectiveness for specific patient groups (effectiveness measures) and the alternative measurement scales and valuations of generic patient well-being (utility measures) such as the Short-Form 36-item General Health Survey Questionnaire ('SF36'), and the Nottingham Health Profile

Box 12.1 Assessment of the value of β-interferon 1b in multiple sclerosis

---

Recombinant β-interferon 1b for relapsing and remitting multiple sclerosis was assessed by the 'quick and clean' health technology assessment approach used by the S&W Development and Evaluation process (Stevens, Colin-Jones, & Gabbay, 1995).
There are six steps in the process:

1. *Define question with key customers*: Health commissions concerned at expensive drug for which benefits seem equivocal or limited.
2. *Literature search* using standard databases, enquiry to experts, references of references.
3. *Tabulation and critical appraisal of data*: at time of assessment, one phase III RCT, a small RCT of intrathecal β-interferon 1b and preliminary unpublished results on β-interferon 1a were available. Critical appraisal of the RCT included the relevance and subjectivity of outcome measures and the patient drop-outs not analysed in the study.
4. *Assessment of benefits and disbenefits*, versus standard therapy.
5. *Assessment of costs and savings* versus standard therapy.
6. *Peer review and presentation of findings* to South and West Development and Evaluation Committee.

Summary of Development and Evaluation Committee report

- β-interferon is one of the first treatments for which there is some evidence of reduction in disease activity in multiple sclerosis (MS). None of the current treatment options prevents relapse or slows progression in MS.
- The prevalence of MS is estimated to be 1:1000 for Southern England, 65% of which (320 people per million population) have the relapse–remitting form of the disease and as such are candidates for the drug.
- Much of the trial evidence emphasised lesions visible on MRI scan. There is inconclusive evidence, that both β-interferon could reduce relapse rates by a third and that β-interferon may have some effect in reducing disease progression.

Box 12.1 *Continued*

- Drug costs alone would be some £10,000 per patient per year. Additional costs would be incurred by the need to check for possible haematological and biochemical abnormalities resulting from drug therapy. Some savings, e.g. hospitalisation costs, would result from a reduction in relapse rate.
- There is currently insufficient clinical evidence of benefit for advocating widespread use of such an expensive drug.

(Adapted from Mortimore, (1996)).

Box 12.2   Levels of outcome in health care assessment

Efficacy	Benefit (from a health care intervention) under ideal conditions.
Effectiveness	Benefit (from a health care intervention) under actual conditions of use.
Cost-Effectiveness	Cost per unit benefit (from a health care intervention), where benefit is measured in units specific to the patient group in question.
Cost-utility	Cost per unit benefit (from a health care intervention), where benefit is measured in generic units, e.g. QALYs which could apply to any patient group.
Impact	The broad effects of a health care intervention assessed for policy purposes.

(Jenkinson, 1994). Some of the latter are potentially particularly valuable in health care priority setting, in that they can be used to generate single index measures (for instance, quality adjusted life years (QALYs) or disability adjusted life years (DALYs)), which facilitate judgements between the value of interventions between different patient groups, i.e. cost-utility analysis. The development of outcomes is a rapidly developing field closely overlapping with the effectiveness revolution but is not elaborated further here (Bowling, 1991, 1995; Jenkinson, 1994).

Cost Measurement

The obverse of outcome measurement is the measurement of cost. Although there has been, and remains, controversy about the relative place of cost-effectiveness as opposed to pure effectiveness arguments in health care decisions, the understanding of scarcity and opportunity cost have put cost-effectiveness measurement centre stage in the effectiveness revolution. The appearance of some very expensive new technologies, particularly pharmaceuticals, e.g. β-interferon, selective serotonin reuptake inhibitors, taxol, Dnase, and imaging techniques, e.g. magnetic resonance imaging, spiral CT, and PET scanning, have particularly sharpened the cost debate. Box 12.1 sets out some of the evidence base on β-interferon's potential use in multiple sclerosis. If β-interferon were to be prescribed for the 40% of multiple sclerosis sufferers for whom it is argued to be indicated, the total annual cost could come to some £400 million, the equivalent of the income of an average sized health authority.

Grading the Evidence

The evidence for effectiveness or otherwise of health care has traditionally come from a variety of different levels of evidence. Two critical features of the effectiveness revolution have been, first, explicitly to judge the quality of the evidence and, secondly, to advocate that it be of the highest quality wherever practicable. A number of hierarchies of evidence are in common use for this purpose. All are very similar, rating RCTs highest, and evidence based on unresearched consensus lowest. A typical scale is set out in Box 12.3. More recent such tables have inserted multiple randomised controlled trials, suitably meta-analysed, at the top, and clashes of opinion (in the absence of evidence) at the bottom. The design of RCTs uniquely in effectiveness research ensures a random, and therefore more probably even, distribution between potential confounders in control and intervention groups. But RCTs are expensive and can have restrictive external validity so that it may not always be possible or even desirable to undertake them. Black (1996) has clarified the situations where this may be so as when RCTs are:

Box 12.3   Grading the evidence on effectiveness

1	Strong evidence obtained from at least one properly designed, randomised controlled trial of appropriate size.
ll-1	Evidence from well-designed controlled trials without randomisation.
ll-2	Evidence from well-designed cohort or case-controlled analytic studies, preferably from more than one centre or research group.
ll-3	Evidence obtained from multiple time series, or from dramatic results in uncontrolled experiments.
lll	Opinions of respected authorities based on clinical evidence, descriptive studies or reports of expert committees.
lV	Evidence inadequate, owing to problems of methodology, e.g. sample size, length or comprehensiveness of follow-up or conflicts of evidence.

(Adapted from the Report of the United States Preventive Services Task Force (Unites States Preventive Services Task Force, 1989).

- unnecessary (for example, in the case of very dramatic observational evidence, such as the effectiveness of smallpox vaccination);
- inappropriate (for example, in the measurement of rare adverse events);
- impossible (for example, where the ethics of randomisation to intensive care might pose an insurmountable barrier); or
- inadequate (for example, where it is crucial to study the effectiveness of an intervention and not merely its efficacy).

Provided its limitations are recognised, there is therefore, a place for observational research, particularly cohort studies which can capitalise on data collected for other purposes. Such studies can be used to help extend the evidence base in concert with RCTs. Another development is the widening of the scope of RCTs from relatively narrow efficacy studies to more pragmatic studies measuring clinical effectiveness in more representative settings and in broader populations than hitherto. And the design of RCTs is increasingly being extended to cover area-wide and even diffuse interventions, where the units of randomisation are practices or whole areas.

Systematic Review of the Evidence

The systematic reviewing of the evidence base therefore searches for evidence in the top grade in preference to lower (and less reliable) levels. But the systematicity of the search is just as important as the ranking of the evidence. Precise rules for how far a search to produce a systematic review has to go have not been universally agreed. The elements of searching can include not just the use of the many electronic databases (e.g. the Cochrane Library, Medline, CINAHL, Psychlit, Science Citation Index) but also hand searching relevant journals and identifying unpublished literature and conference proceedings (Centre for Reviews and Dissemination, 1996). The principle underlying the systematicity of searching is the avoidance of bias. The absence of a systematic search can be a sign of a review setting out to prove a point rather than to appraise the evidence — a common feature of traditional reviews and editorials. Even when reviews have an unbiased intent, a systematic and comprehensive search is necessary because of the bias that can arise when studies with positive or dramatic findings are more likely to be published than those with negative or unexciting results. This 'publication bias' may be more of a problem with smaller studies. The importance of reviews being systematic was underlined by the startling findings of Antman and colleagues (see Table 12.1) (Antman et al., 1992). They compared the conclusions of unsystematic and systematic reviews about treatments for myocardial infarction. As discussed earlier they found a marked delay in the incorporation of findings from RCTs into current wisdom, clearly showing the dangers that can arise when researchers and clinicians fail to synthesise evidence reliably.

Critical Appraisal

Critical appraisal is not new: it has long been of concern to journal editors (who receive, appraise and publish/reject) and to researchers (who find, appraise and synthesise). It has now become a core skill for those planning to use evidence to support health care decisions (who must search, appraise and act). Once the evidence has been sought, the underlying principles of critical appraisal concern the validity and applicability of the research discernible from published papers.

Numerous checklists have been developed to inform critical appraisal both for primary research and review articles (see Box 12.4). Judgements will always be subjective to an extent and critical reviewing may benefit from there being two or more simultaneous reviewers.

Box 12.4   Critical appraisal questions for a review

Ten questions to help you make sense of a review

A   Are the results of the review valid?

    1. Did the review address a clearly focused issue?
    2   Did the authors look for the appropriate sort of papers?
    3   Do you think the important, relevant studies were included?
    4   Did the review's authors do enough to assess the quality of the included studies?
    5   If the results of the review have been combined, was it reasonable to do so?

B   What are the results?

    6   What is the overall result of the review?
    7   How precise are the results?

C   Will the results help locally?

    8   Can the results be applied to the local population?
    9   Were all important outcomes considered?
    10 Are the benefits worth the harms and costs?

(Source: Critical Appraisal Skills Programme, (1996)).

Integrating the Evidence

Integrating evidence from different sources is an essential feature of systematic reviews, whether they are reviews of trials, observational studies, cost-effectiveness analyses or qualitative research. The combining of evidence from multiple different studies is at its most straightforward when the studies are all high-quality RCTs. Here the synthesis can use meta-analysis in which the results of trials are quantitatively reanalysed collectively, ideally using original patient data. It is possible for non-RCTs to be meta-analysed too, but because it is important not to contaminate better studies with poorer ones this is less frequently appropriate. At the very least, however, summarising involves the tabulation of the features of comparable studies, i.e. including design objectives, target population, sample size (intervention and control group), outcomes measured, results and critique.

Interpretation and Delivery of the Evidence

The scale and complexity of the evidence base of health care is vast, requiring both primary research (where the unit of analysis is the patient, the professional, etc.) and secondary research (where the unit of analysis is the primary study). In addition, it needs to be interpreted and delivered to the user in a meaningful and valued form, which means that the scope of secondary research needs to extend beyond systematic reviews of the effectiveness of single interventions. A number of initiatives that have evolved to meet this need for interpretation and delivery are outlined in the next section: these include tertiary reviews of, disease-wide topics, guidelines, new information facilities, and dissemination initiatives. The delivery of information, whether primary research direct, systematic reviews or further interpretative reviews is becoming an important area of research, covering not only delivery systems but also the receptivity of the target audience.

The example in Table 12.1 of the failure to systematically review the evidence also points to the barriers to uptake of new findings. One is the reliance on personal experience rather than evidence. The problem with personal experience is that it can favour visible but possibly unimportant findings (such as the apparent control of arrhythmias with antiarrhythmic drugs), over less immediate but vital findings (such as longer-term mortality prevented by thrombolytics). Such 'dissemination' issues seem destined to become a central concern of the effectiveness revolution, and one in which public health practitioners have the key role to play.

INITIATIVES IN EVIDENCE-BASED HEALTH CARE

Introduction

There are already a number of excellent guides to initiatives in evidence-based health care which are not repeated here.[3] Instead, below is a selected list of key UK initiatives in effectiveness and evidence-based health care. Public health practitioners have been particularly involved in all of them, and they have been selected on the basis of what they illustrate about the role of public health in this field. The initiatives are grouped for convenience in terms of the barriers to evidence-based health care that each tackles, although Table 12.2 shows that many of the initiatives straddle more than one of these barriers.

- lack of availability of relevant high quality information;
- lack of access to relevant high quality information;
- inadequate skills in finding, appraising and acting on evidence;
- barriers in the organisation of work or care.

Overcoming the lack of availability of relevant high quality information

NHS R&D Strategy

The NHS Research & Development strategy was launched in 1991, following a House of Lords report on Priorities in Medical Research (House of Lords, 1988). The report noted an imbalance in the allocation of research funds, with much spent on biomedical research but too little on health service issues. The aim of the R&D strategy, therefore, as set out by the first Director of Research and Development, Professor Michael Peckham, was to create a 'research based health service in which reliable and relevant information is available for decisions on health policy, clinical practice and the management of services' (Peckham, 1993). The six functions of the R&D strategy are:

- identifying NHS requirements for knowledge;
- ensuring that the knowledge required is produced;
- disseminating research based information;

---

[3] For instance, the SCHARR guide to evidence-based practice, available both on the World Wide Web (http://www.shef.ac.uk/uni/academic/R-Z/scharr/ir/netting.html)

Table 12.2 Summary of initiatives

Barrier	Initiatives	Specific public health feature
Lack of availability of relevant high quality information	NHS R&D strategy HTA programme	Starting with the needs of the NHS for information
	Cochrane Collaboration Centre for Reviews and Dissemination	Systematic reviews take a 'population approach' to evidence
	South and West Development and Evaluation Service (DEC); and similar initiatives	Cost-utility analysis with clear purchaser/public health audience
	Health Care Needs Assessment series	Covers three issues relevant to service planners for entire disease groups: current provision, burden of disease, cost-effectiveness
Lack of access to relevant high quality information	Cochrane Library	Brings together systematic reviews, with clinical outcomes, that pass certain quality standards
	National Research Register	Access to the population of research going on within the NHS
	Aggressive Research Intelligence Facility	A regional information service targeted at the special needs of purchasers and public health practitioners
	GEARS	A local database targeted at the special needs of purhasers and public health practitioners
Inadequate skills in finding, appraising and acting on evidence	Critical Appraisal Skills Programme	Critical appraisal skills developed in 'non-tribal' ways
	Getting Research into Practice and Purchasing (GRiPP)	Population approach to change
Barriers in the organisation of work or care	Guidelines	Multi-disciplinary, population approach
	PACE	Moving clinical effectiveness from 'project to main stream'
	DEC	Linking reports to cost-effectiveness to recommendations for action
	GRiPP	'Whole system' approach to change

THE EFFECTIVENESS REVOLUTION AND PUBLIC HEALTH   217

- promoting the use of R&D findings;
- promoting an evaluative culture;
- developing and evaluating the R&D strategy.

HTA Programme

The R&D strategy has a number of programmes for funding research, both nationally and regionally. One of the national programmes is the Health Technology Assessment (HTA) programme[4], which aims 'to ensure that high quality research information on the costs, effectiveness and broader impact of health technologies is produced in the most efficient way for those who use, manage and work in the NHS' (Department of Health, 1996). The programme takes a broad view of 'health technologies' to cover all health care interventions, across the whole spectrum of medical, nursing and health practice. It spends some £5 million per year on research, has to date identified over 250 evaluation questions of importance to the health service and has funded nearly 100 research projects to help answer these questions. Funding is split between new primary research, usually randomised controlled trials, and secondary research reviews, usually systematic reviews[5]. The first completed reviews were published in 1997 and included screening for prostate cancer using prostate specific antigen (not supported by the evidence) and near-patient testing in general practice. Some of the trials are on topics such as stroke rehabilitation, surgery for back pain and counselling for mental health problems.

Cochrane Collaboration

This is an international endeavour in which people from many different countries systematically find, appraise and review available evidence from randomised controlled trials about the effects of health care. The Collaboration aims to develop and maintain systematic, up-to-date reviews of RCTs of all forms of health care and to make this information readily available to clinicians and other

---

[4] The HTA programme is co-ordinated from the National Co-ordinating Centre (NCCHTA), a collaboration between the Wessex Institute for Health Research and Development at Southhampton University and health care groups at York University
[5] Currently, most systematic reviews deal with single interventions or with narrow group of interventions. Secondary research can of course go much wider than this to include reviews which deal with service delivery or patterns of care, as well as those in which the main focus is to model the costs and effectiveness of interventions

decision makers at all levels of health care systems. The UK Cochrane Centre opened in Oxford in 1992.

Centre for Reviews and Dissemination

The NHS Centre for Reviews and Dissemination (CRD) in York produces and disseminates reviews of the effectiveness and cost-effectiveness of health care interventions. These reviews are published as CRD reports, Effective Health Care Bulletins, and Effectiveness Matters reports. In addition, the Centre maintains two public databases, the Database of Abstracts of Reviews and Effectiveness (DARE) and the NHS Economic Evaluation Database. Both are available on the Internet and through dial-up access. DARE is also available as part of the Cochrane Library.

Development and Evaluation Service (South & West Region)

South & West's Development and Evaluation service is based on a partnership between four players in the cost-effectiveness field: health authorities and other decision makers, who identify the questions of concern; the Wessex Institute for Health Research & Development, which produces 'quick and clean' reports on the question; the Regional Development and Evaluation Committee, which makes recommendations on the basis of the reports; and the Regional Research and Development Directorate, which funds the service (Stevens et al., 1995). Each DEC report summarises existing evidence in such a way as to generate sufficiently clear cost and effectiveness calculations to allow a recommendation on local use. Partnerships with similar objectives have been set up in other parts of the UK, including Scotland (Scottish Health Purchasing Information Centre) and Trent (Trent DEC). Each of these initiatives has demonstrated a capacity to provide vital information at short notice where necessary, as in the case of the South and West DEC and Trent reports on β-interferon for Multiple Sclerosis (see Table 12.2).

Health Care Needs Assessment series

The Health Care Needs Assessment series comprises some 28 disease or service-wide reviews. Each review is intended to inform purchasers of health care of the key elements of the health care needs of a typical population. These key elements comprise prevalence, service effectiveness and current service pattern. The reviews were sponsored by the Department of Health's 'District Health Authority Project' following the NHS review of 1990; and were published as three volumes (two in 1994 and one in 1997) made directly available to purchasers of health (Stevens & Raftery, 1994, 1997)[6].

Overcoming the lack of access to relevant high quality information

Cochrane Library

The Cochrane Library (an electronic, not paper library) is the chief product of the Cochrane Collaboration and an unrivalled source of high quality evidence about the effects of health care. It currently contains five resources: the Cochrane Database of Systematic Reviews; CRD's Database of Abstracts of Reviews of Effectiveness; the Cochrane Reviews Methodology Database; the Cochrane Controlled Trials Register; and information about the Cochrane Collaboration. It runs on personal computers, is updated four times a year and is not expensive. Every public health practitioner should have ready access to a copy.

Aggressive Research Intelligence Facility (ARIF)

The West Midlands Aggressive Research Intelligence Facility was set up in 1996 principally to maintain and make available hard copies of systematic reviews to west Midlands purchasers. ARIF responds to searches for evidence from its clients by supplying and discussing and interpreting the review and the strategy for obtaining further evidence.

GEARS

Getting Easier Access to Reviews (GEARS) is a database designed to meet the immediate information needs of public health practitioners. Funded by the health authorities in South & West, it brings together two sorts of reviews or summaries: those that are methodologically rigorous (but for various reasons would not be on the Cochrane Library), and those that are 'politically' important (such as Royal College or King's Fund reports). The hope is that a quick search on GEARS will provide the five or ten key references needed, either to arm the searcher for an imminent meeting, or as preparation for a more extensive familiarisation with the literature.

---

[6] A third series and an updating of the first series are currently under discussion.

GEARS is therefore designed to be used in conjunction with the more extensive resources described above.

The National Research Register (NRR)

The national research register is a centrally resourced database of research in the NHS that has been (or is about to be) funded. It uses a co-ordinated network of PC-based project registers to enable information to be regularly updated.

Overcoming the problem of inadequate skills in finding, appraising and acting on evidence

Critical Appraisal Skills Programme (CASP)

CASP is a programme, based in Anglia and Oxford, but working across the whole of the UK, that aims to help decision-makers develop skills in the critical appraisal of evidence about effectiveness, in order to promote the delivery of evidence based health care (Critical Appraisal Skills Programme, 1996). The major components of CASP are a programme of workshops, a central support team, a training the trainer programme, a growing support network of enthusiastic people and an evolving programme of development and evaluation. Fundamental principles for CASP include: workshops should be multi-disciplinary; skills in organising and delivering workshops should be cascaded as widely as possible; learning should be problem-based and enjoyable; and all teaching should be interactive.

Overcoming barriers in the organisation of work or care

Clinical Guidelines

Clinical guidelines of varying thoroughness have long existed, but are gaining new accuracy, and in the USA in particular, are often now based on systematic reviews. The difference is one of emphasis first towards making practice recommendations, and second towards clinical problem solving. The latter means that a particular guideline although perhaps covering a single clinical concern often covers a short sequence of decisions. The Department of Health has supported several of the UK's Colleges and professional bodies to take the lead (NHS Executive, 1996) and many of these are taking a fully evidence-based approach, basing their guidelines on a systematic review of research,. A typical example is the forthcoming Royal College of Psychiatrists' Guideline on 'The management of violence in clinical settings' (J. Wing, 1997, personal communication). The key criteria for successful guidelines have been set out by Russell and Grimshaw (Grimshaw & Russell, 1993). They need to be not only clear, valid, reproducible, reliable, cost-effective, and clinically applicable, but also representative, flexible, reviewable and amenable to clinical audit.

GRiPP

GRiPP (Getting Research into Practice and Purchasing) is a system designed to achieve evidence-supported change in the four counties of Berkshire, Buckinghamshire, Oxfordshire and Northamptonshire. Priorities are set by health authority chief executives, and topics currently in hand include neurosciences, breast cancer, colorectal cancers, gynaecological cancers and lung cancer. The system consists of the following components: (i) evidence gathering, appraisal and synthesis, undertaken on a collaborative basis between the four counties; (ii) the development of guidelines and appropriate information for purchasers and the public, led by one of the four counties; (iii) implementation of the guidelines and information locally; (iv) audit of the impact of these, undertaken collaboratively among the four counties.

Promoting Action on Clinical Effectiveness (PACE)

PACE is a King's Fund programme funded by the NHS Executive to demonstrate the effective implementation of evidence-based practice and identify the factors for success. It networks local projects: two from each NHS region in England. Each project is based either on health authority or trust or sometimes (preferably) on a partnership of the two. Each covers a single topic (e.g. stroke prevention, *H. pylori* eradication, family support for schizophrenia) determined by the existence of usable and clear evidence. Each seeks to build on existing key facilities such as intelligence (library) services, local audit programmes or professional education, and to align them to carry forward a proposed evidence-based change.

CONCLUSIONS

There are Limits to Rationality

The converging strands of cost-effectiveness analysis, health technology assessment and evidence-based medicine have contributed to enormous changes in the planning and delivery of health care in the United Kingdom and elsewhere. These changes, in which public health practitioners have played a prominent part, certainly merit the title 'effectiveness revolution'. At the same time, we must recognise that the use of effectiveness (or cost-effectiveness or appropriateness) information by public health practitioners can be problematic (Milne & Hicks, 1996), for several reasons.

First, there are still enormous gaps in the evidence, both about a population's health problems and about the appropriateness of services available to help those problems. Secondly, even when we know a lot, evidence can only at best be one part of a decision about the provision of services. It is proper that other factors should play a part (Fig. 12.2): the views of patients, their representatives or the community; the views of professionals in the area; and top-down instructions, whether from the NHS Executive or elsewhere. The difficulty lies in reconciling the tensions from these different influences, particularly in situations where even compelling evidence can easily be ignored. Applying the evidence to the millions of complex clinical and planning decisions taken each year in the NHS is seldom easy or comfortable. It always requires effort, usually has 'resource implications' and frequently provokes antagonism.

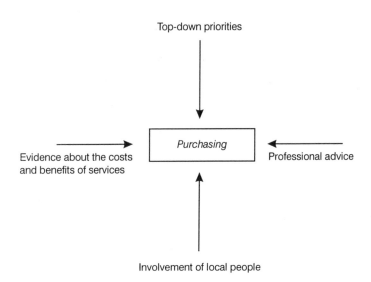

Fig. 12.2 Factors influencing purchasing decisions. (Adapted from Cochrane *et al.*, 1991.)

What About the Rest of Public Health Practice?

Some are concerned that the effectiveness revolution is distorting the practice of public health, distracting scarce time and resources from what should be our overriding concern to improve the health of the population. There are parallel concerns that the close involvement of public health practitioners in the UK since the NHS reforms with the new commissioning function may distract from other, possibly more compelling (though perhaps not more cost-effective) ways of improving the public health.

Such concerns must be taken seriously. At the same time, we must also remember that the effectiveness revolution has important messages for all public health practitioners: not just those working to help develop clinical practice, but also those working in communicable disease control, health promotion, intersectoral work and so on. There are lessons for us all in terms of the effectiveness and cost-effectiveness or our own practice, of the methods we use to bring about health-promoting changes in society. We cannot advocate cost-effectiveness for others and exempt ourselves: we need to become part of the evidence-based culture.

A Final Word...

The effectiveness revolution has generated some valuable aphorisms. We must never forget that 'absence of evidence is not evidence of absence'. We must beware of dismissing the unproven as ineffective and we must seek cost-effective solutions to problems of cost-effectiveness. For the effectiveness revolution is surely here to stay, which means that we must advocate evidence-based practice by others (clinicians, politicians, advertisers, whoever) and that we must practise it ourselves (by thinking critically and looking for the best evidence about how we work). When in ten years' time we look back on the 20th anniversary of the publication of the Acheson report, we will see that things have changed for good: that public health practitioners – however, and wherever, they work — consider far more than they ever used to the questions: Does it work? And is it worth it?

REFERENCES

Antman E, Lau J, Kupelnick B, Mosteller F, Chalmers T 1992 A comparison of results of meta-analyses of randomized control trials and recommendations of experts. Journal of the American Medical Association, 268: 240–8

Black N 1996 Why we need observational studies to evaluate the effectiveness of health care. British Medical Journal, 312: 1215–18

Bowling A 1991 Measuring Health. Milton Keynes: Open University

Bowling A 1995 Measuring Disease. Milton Keynes: Open University

Centre for Reviews and Dissemination 1996 Undertaking systematic reviews of research on effectiveness. CRD guidelines for those carrying out or commissioning reviews. NHS Centre for Reviews and Dissemination.

Cochrane A 1972 Effectiveness and Efficiency: Random reflections on the health service. Leeds: Nuffield Provincial Hospitals Trust

Cochrane M, Ham C, Heginbotham C, Smith R 1991 Rationing: at the cutting edge. British Medical Journal, 303: 1039–42

Committee of Enquiry into the Future of the Public Health Function 1988 Public Health in England. The report of the committee of inquiry into the future development of the public health function.

Critical Appraisal Skills Programme 1996 Orientation Guide. Oxford: Institute of Health Sciences

Department of Health 1996 Standing Group on Health Technology Annual Report. Department of Health

DHA Project 1991 Anonymous. Assessing health care needs. Department of Health.

Donabedian A 1973 Aspects of Medical Care Administration. Specifying requirements for health care. Cambridge, MA: Harvard

Drummond MF 1993 The contribution of health economics to cost-effective health care delivery. In Purchasing and Providing Cost-effective Health Care. ed. Drummond MF, Maynard A, London: Churchill Livingstone

Evidence Based Medicine Working Group 1992 Evidence-Based Medicine. Journal of the American Medical Association, 268: 2420–5

Grimshaw J, Russell I 1993 Achieving health gain through clinical guidelines. I: Developing scientifically valid guidelines. Quality in Health Care 2: 243–8

Ham C 1996 The future of the NHS. British Medical Journal, 313: 1277–8

House of Lords 1988 Priorities in Medical Research. London: HMSO

Illich I 1976 Limits to Medicine. Marion Boyers

Jenkinson C ed. 1994 Measuring Health and Medical Outcomes. London: UCL Press

McKeown T 1979 The Role of Medicine. Oxford: Blackwell

Milne R, Hicks N 1996 EBM Notebook: evidence-based purchasing. Evidence-Based Medicine 1: 101–2

Mooney GH 1986 Economics, Medicine and Health Care. Brighton: Wheatsheaf

Mortimore A 1996 Interferon beta therapy for multiple sclerosis. In Health Technology Evaluation Research Reviews III. ed Stevens A, Winchester: Wessex Institute of Public Health Medicine

NHS Executive 1996 Clinical guidelines: using guidelines to improve patient care in the NHS. NHS Executive.

Peckham M 1993 Research for Health. Department of Health

Robinson R 1996 The impact of the NHS reforms 1991–1995: a review of research evidence. Journal of Public Health Medicine 18: 337–42

Sackett D, Rosenberg W, Gray J, Haynes R, Richardson W 1996 Evidence based medicine: what it is and what it isn't. British Medical Journal, 312: 71–2

Secretaries of State for Health, Wales, Northern Ireland and Scotland 1989 Working for Patients. London: Department of Health

Stevens A, Colin-Jones D, Gabbay J 1995 'Quick and clean': authoritative health technology assessment for local health care contracting. Health Trends 27: 37–42

Stevens A, Gabbay J 1991 Needs assessment needs assessment. Health Trends 23: 20–3

Stevens A, Raftery J 1994 Health Care Needs Assessment. Abingdon, Oxon: Radcliffe Medical Press

Stevens A, Raftery J 1997 Health Care Needs Assessment. Second Series. Abingdon, Oxon: Radcliffe Medical Press

United States Preventive Services Task Force 1989 Guide to clinical preventive services. An assessment of 169 interventions. Williams and Williams.

US Congress Office of Technology Assessment 1994 Identifying health technologies that work: searching for the evidence. US Government Printing Office.

Wennberg JE, Freeman JL, Culp WJ 1987 Are hospital services rationed in New Haven or over-utilised in Boston? Lancet i: 1185–9

Wyatt J 1991 Use and sources of medical knowledge. Lancet 338: 1368–73

13. Quality in Healthcare: A public health perspective

Liam Donaldson and David Benton

INTRODUCTION

The public health perspective is most often that of the health of populations. This means attention being directed towards those health problems which do not necessarily apply to people receiving medical care nor to those which are amenable to clinical intervention. However, for a number of reasons the concerns of a modern public health function must also be with the care of patients. First, the health of the population can be improved by health services delivered to patients, albeit to a much more limited extent than through the wider health strategies which are described in other chapters of this book. Secondly, as the population ages, as the prevalence of chronic diseases increases, and as new therapies create opportunities to maintain people who might otherwise have died, the pool of patients in the population will increase. Thirdly, in Britain and many other countries, those with public health expertise are increasingly employed by health services and so it is inevitable that their skills will be sought in decisions concerning the organisation and delivery of health services as well as in wider health issues.

The outcome of the care received by patients is therefore of importance to the public health. This chapter addresses the issues in the broad context of quality in health care. This is a large and complex field in which ideas, opinions, schools of thought, knowledge and practical experience co-exist but seldom converge. Much of the early methodological work on health care quality was undertaken in North America where the devolved and diverse medical care arrangements meant that it was difficult to find applications implemented across the whole system of care. This remains the case although there are many broad-ranging quality improvement programmes which have been applied to parts of the health care system in the United States. Some of these are impressive and usually further advanced than those in most European countries in the strength of their conceptual frameworks and in their degree of innovation. Good examples can be found in the work of the Joint Commission on Accreditation of Health Care Organisations (JCAHO, 1989).

In Britain, until the end of the 1980s, the predominant philosophy of quality improvement was professionally-based. A long tradition of involvement in peer review within particular clinical disciplines has been led by the medical Royal Colleges whilst a small number of pioneering multi-disciplinary programmes have concentrated on exploring the causes of particular adverse outcomes of care such as maternal or perioperative deaths. In addition, work on the use of standard setting as part of an action research approach has been developed by Kitson *et al.* (1990) in the Royal College of Nursing's Standards of Care Project.

In the late 1980s and early 1990s, this professionally driven philosophy changed as a consequence of the reforms of the British National Health Service introduced at that time. Out of this process of reform, in Britain, came a belief that the design of the health care system itself could be a driving force for quality improvement. With it, also, came new processes of accountability for health care professionals for the quality of care they delivered. So too, came a move towards viewing patients more as consumers of health care with rights, entitlements and access to information on the quality of care they should expect to receive.

However, despite three decades of research and analysis, fundamental questions remain about health care quality: what is it? how is it defined? how is it measured? how is it improved? In this chapter, trends in the evolution of thinking about quality in health care are discussed in the context of concepts and philosophies, mechanisms of quality improvement, and methods for evaluating it.

CONCEPTS

Many definitions have sought to encapsulate the concept of quality in health care. These have been diverse in their origins ranging from the perspectives of professional bodies, through researchers seeking to establish conceptual frameworks, to those who seek to draw parallels between health care and quality philosophies which have been successful in international companies.

The concept of quality which has been most enduring in health care is that first put forward in the mid-1960s by the North American health services researcher, Avedis Donabedian (Donabedian, 1966). This proposed a meaning for quality of health care, and a way of evaluating it in three related components: structural (the physical features of health care such as buildings, equipment, staff); process (how facilities and resources are used to diagnose and treat patients); and, outcome (the impact of care on a patient's health status). Donabedian has developed his classification further over the years, for example, introducing additional practical elements to the conceptualisation of health care quality such as: the 'goodness' of technical care, the 'goodness' of interpersonal relationships between those providing care and patients; and, 'goodness' of the amenities of care (Donabedian, 1989).

Donabedian's work on quality of health care has been very influential over the years and is still widely quoted. It remains particularly helpful in providing a framework for thinking through, and debating, quality issues. There are few examples of it being used systematically within health services in the fields of policy-making, management, information systems or evaluation. One within Britain is The Royal College of Nursing's 'Standards of Care' project and the subsequent 'Dynamic Standard Setting System' developed by Kitson et al. (1990). Areas as diverse as rheumatic disease, management in nursing, family planning and paediatrics have all been addressed. It does, however, seem surprising that the Donabedian framework has not been exploited more widely. To assess a service by seeking to understand what resources are being deployed (structures), how they are used (processes) and to what end (outcomes) has enormous appeal in simplicity and clarity. It is also easy to communicate to staff and has a basis in common-sense. The explanation for the lack of routine use of the Donabedian framework of structures, processes and outcomes is perhaps that less attention has been given to exploring the dynamics and the way in which the three components inter-relate. Rather, the debate has centred on the individual elements which have come to be seen, inappropriately, in hierarchical terms. Thus, outcome is viewed by many as the prime concern in health care quality whilst the structural aspect has been denigrated and is seen as less meaningful.

Whilst the real issues are, indeed, in the inter-relationship (neither structure, process nor outcome should be seen in isolation), ironically, in certain circumstances a focus on the structural aspect of quality can be very valuable. This is particularly so, when an area of service is grossly underdeveloped. For example, in a part of a country with no physicians or other staff with expertise in the care of diabetes mellitus, it is likely that services for that group of the population would be of poorer quality than in an area where such resources are available. Of course, there are then important questions about how the resources are used in the care of diabetic people (the process aspect of quality), but a first step-up in quality of care is likely to be achieved through ensuring that adequate staff are in place with the proper training and with access to facilities.

Many who have sought to develop definitions and measures of quality within health services have regarded outcome as the holy grail. Attention to outcomes of care has a long history. A particular landmark in North America is the work of Ernest Codman in Massachusetts in the early part of the present century (Codman, 1914). Codman, a surgeon, recognised the importance of using aggregated clinical data in making judgements about the quality of care and the scope for its improvement. He classified errors of surgical treatment into one of four categories as due to: lack of technical knowledge or skill, lack of surgical judgement, lack of care or equipment or lack of diagnostic skill. His 'end-result' philosophy was shunned by influential bodies at the time as the ideas of many pioneers in the history of public health have been. He started his own hospital so that he could continue to practice his philosophy. Today, Codman's work is seen as a beacon of early enlightenment in the quality of care movement. In Britain, many public health historians have drawn attention to the insight of Florence Nightingale. In addition to being the founder of modern nursing, and a hospital and social reformer, Miss Nightingale was also described as the 'passionate statistician'. On her return from the Crimean War, she sought to create a system to gather data on hospital patients in which she would examine mortality from different causes in different hospitals. Her scheme for Uniform Hospital Statistics was acclaimed at the International Statistical Congress held in London in the summer of 1860.

Within the modern outcomes field a number of themes can be recognised. The use of adverse outcomes has been used to draw conclusions about quality. The importance of the sentinel event was promoted by Rutstein and his colleagues (Rutstein et al., 1976) who argued that the measurement of quality often failed because of the difficulty in defining and assessing different degrees of health. The less ambiguous concept of unnecessary death, disease or disability was seen as a warning that quality needed to be improved and the analogy with other disaster investigations was drawn by Rutstein in the use of the metaphor for his work: 'airplane crashes in health'. In Britain, the approach was developed and implemented in the National Health Service with the creation of a new body of routine data on so-called avoidable deaths. This was analysed and presented by geographical area (Charlton *et al.*, 1983).

Reacting to, or seeking out, adverse outcomes of care is a necessary process when there are serious lapses in the standard of health care provided. The resulting investigation has its focus on establishing the facts, identifying the possible contributory factors and formulating action to be taken to try to avoid a repetition. With a major incident, an enquiry with findings and recommendations will often lead to new policy-making and legislation which affect a whole health service not just the institution which was the subject of the problems. Reacting to adverse events in this way is important as part of an overall quality programme and is part of the proper process of public accountability. Despite the numbers of inquiries that do take place (for example, into homicides involving mentally ill people), lessons are not routinely learned and implemented by services that have not been directly involved in the event (Blain & Donaldson, 1995).

In the past, much of the focus in thinking about outcomes has been on clinical measures such as mortality or complications of treatment and biochemical or haematological indices. Increasingly, there is a recognition that outcome must be viewed more widely and also encompass dimensions, such as the psychological impact of medical care, quality of life of patients and their carers as well as patients' own views on the care received.

With this broader conceptualisation of outcome of care, an important element of quality becomes the extent to which different treatments or other interventions, in fact, do improve the outcome of patients' care. This aspect of quality has been a field of study in its own right. Three separate concepts are relevant – efficacy, effectiveness, and appropriateness (Hopkins, 1993). Efficacy is the ability of an intervention to produce a desired outcome in ideal conditions. Thus, a statement on efficacy of a treatment may be made after concluding a large randomised controlled trial. However, the application of the same treatment in day-to-day practice will not result in it having a uniform and consistent impact on outcome. How an intervention 'performs' is thus its effectiveness. How effective it is depends on a wide range of factors including the skill and training of the health care professional administering it, the nature of the patient population, the institution in which it is delivered.

Repeatedly, observations have been made on the occurrence of wide variation in medical practice within different populations or between different services. Such variations can have multiple causes but because they have often been shown not to be due to justifiable differences in morbidity, the idea of 'appropriateness' has become an important element of discussions on defining quality in health care. The meaning of appropriateness has been reviewed by Hopkins (1993) who has distinguished between the professional perspective, the lay perspective and the perspective of society as a whole in deciding what is appropriate and what is not in health care. A good example of the complexity of these issues is the case of hysterectomy (Lilford, 1997) an intervention subject to widespread variation between countries, within countries and between social and occupational groups.

Given the complexity of these concepts, and their inter-relationships, it may be helpful to redefine them through these simple questions: 'what is the right thing to do?' (efficacy); 'are we doing the right thing?' (appropriateness); 'are we doing the right thing right?' (effectiveness). Finally, it is important to recognise the relevance of financial resources to discussions about this aspect of quality. Concepts such as cost-effectiveness are increasingly important to health services working with finite resources in an environment of rapidly rising demand.

A further perspective on health care quality emerges if it is recognised that relying wholly on a strategy of quality improvement based upon addressing problems as they arise is inappropriate. This has been referred to by Berwick (1989) as an approach which concentrates on the 'bad apples'. Berwick (1989) sets this in a public health context by pointing out that dealing with the tail of a (normal-type) distribution is not as effective as shifting the whole curve (say) to the left (the hypothetical direction of improvement).

Berwick's concept of quality is important because it is partly derived from, and builds a bridge between, health care quality and industrial quality improvement philosophies. The latter called variously total quality management or continuous quality improvement involve orientating the whole company or organisation to a quality philosophy. The precise approach will differ according to who has originated it but many have common features: leadership from the top of the organisation; empowerment of staff; team work; prevention (rather than simply correction) of adverse outcomes;

analysing, simplifying and improving processes; and, a strong customer focus. One of the early proponents of total quality management was W. Edwards Deming an American. Born in 1900, a graduate in engineering and mathematical statistics, he became interested in statistical control of industrial process. Deming travelled to post-war Japan and lectured to Japanese industrialists on his emerging theory of total quality management as a recipe for commercial success. Key to Deming's ideas was a process which he called a 'chain reaction' — taking measures to prevent defects in manufacture leads to lower costs which leads to higher productivity and quality which leads to a greater market share because of better quality at lower prices (Deming, 1986). This message was particularly well received by Japanese industry at the time which had a reputation for producing poor quality goods. The principles of total quality management or continuous quality improvement in various different forms have been introduced by the industrial and service sectors in most industrialised countries. The applicability of these concepts to health care has been recognised for some time but they are still not in widespread use.

Other concepts of quality have sought to identify different dimensions as part of a framework. Some, in particular, have also addressed the population aspects. A World Health Organisation working group on quality (World Health Organisation, 1989) identified four components: performance, resource use, risk management and patient satisfaction. When Maxwell in the mid-1980s identified a lack of progress over several decades in conceptualising health care quality, he proposed six dimensions of quality: access to services, relevance to need (for the whole community), effectiveness (for individual patients), equity, social acceptability, efficiency (Maxwell, 1984). The incorporation of a population dimension makes the Maxwell classification of quality particularly useful for the British National Health Service. Indeed, over a decade later, echoes of it are to be found within the service's current strategic documents (Secretary of State For Health, 1996). However, like Donabedian's formulation, its principal use has been in shaping debate and informing strategy rather than in routine management and evaluation of services.

Quality can also be seen as a concept which is embodied within the design of the system of health care itself and the features which influence it can be described. This will differ from country to country. In Britain, when reforms to the National Health Service were introduced in 1990, the operation of the service was re-designed. A fundamental feature of the new system was the separation of responsibility for the purchasing of care from its provision. Thus, health authorities and some general practitioners (general practice fundholders) were allocated funds to meet the health needs of local populations. Services were delivered as a result of contracts agreed between these bodies and those responsible for the provision of services, organisations called NHS Trusts (hospitals and/or community health service providers). The resulting internal market for public health care in Britain could be seen as creating three potential forces which would improve quality as the system operated: (a) competition between NHS Trusts for a share of available resources would be on the basis of quality as well as cost, tending to drive up quality as hospitals sought to out-perform each other; (b) purchaser choice as health authorities and general practitioners sought to place contracts in places where the services were best; and, (c) contract specification as health authorities and general practitioners sought to agree the basis for improvement in quality through placing clauses in contracts for services.

In reviewing the concepts which make up the field of health care quality, it is striking how many different perspectives co-exist. Thus, a person might ask the seemingly simple question, 'how good is our health care?'. Such a question could be taken to be posing a whole series of questions such as: 'how appropriate is our health care?' 'how clinically effective is it?' 'how does it influence outcomes which are relevant to patients and their carers?' 'how does it influence outcomes which health care professionals have demonstrated as the most clinically meaningful?' 'how good on organisation are we?' 'what systems are in place to ensure that there is continuous improvement of the processes of care?' 'How many adverse outcomes of care occur and how do we ensure that future patients benefit from investigations of them?'

Posing the questions demonstrates that none of these questions can be discarded as irrelevant. Different perspectives on quality are necessary depending on the service, and the level of the organisation from which the issues are being viewed.

MECHANISMS

A wide variety of ways exist to bring about improvements in quality of care. In this section, they are addressed in three broad categories: those which are mediated through professional practice, those which require an organisational approach and measures to empower patients. The categories are not mutually exclusive.

Improving Professional Practice

Ensuring the delivery of high quality care to patients has been embodied within the ethos of all health care professions. Less consistency and certainty has attended attempts to make more explicit the assessment of the quality of professional practice, the introduction of quality assurance methods or ensuring that the scope for improvement is recognised and acted upon. There is little doubt that mechanisms directed towards raising standards of clinical practice are a vital part of strategies for quality improvement. However, which mechanisms are best for achieving change in particular circumstances is more difficult to determine.

Examining standards of practice using peer review has a long tradition in medicine (Lembcke, 1967), less so in other health professions. In Britain, in the past, much of the leadership has come either from the Royal Colleges or from a small number of pioneering clinical departments. This rather inconsistent approach changed with the requirement for all doctors to participate in medical audit when the 1990 National Health Service reforms were introduced. Soon after the concept was broadened to involve other health care professions (clinical audit). These forms of audit are a process of cyclical standard setting (Fig. 13.1) which involve critically examining present practice, setting criteria for improvement based on best practice information, implementing change and checking to see that improvement has taken place.

Looking at standard-setting more broadly, five professionally based quality improvement methods in common use incorporate standards (Irvine & Donaldson, 1993): critical incident review (clinical team members review adverse outcomes such as case fatality or complications); critical event monitoring (similar to critical incident review by collecting and aggregating data over time to allow trends to be examined); confidential enquiries (such as those into maternal or perioperative deaths); random clinical record review (involving peer group discussion of records of individual cases); criteria-based review (the development of explicit criteria and standards for the diagnosis investigation and management of patients with specific diseases and standards and assessing a clinician's performance against those).

Fundamental to improving the quality of care provided to

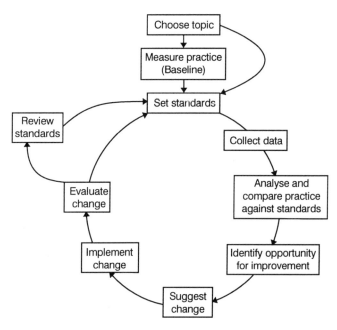

Fig. 13.1 The professional audit cycle. (Source: Donaldson & Donaldson, 1993.)

patients by health care professionals is ensuring that the knowledge derived from research is rapidly adopted into practice. It is widely acknowledged that this is not generally the case, for example: 'the profession has placed value on developing the basic science of medicine; it has not emphasised the process by which science is translated into practice' (Eddy, 1982). This failure of transference of research findings into routine practice has been demonstrated in numerous clinical fields. For example, the failure of widespread adoption of antenatal corticosteroids in appropriate cases as a cheap and effective alternative to surfactants and neonatal intensive care (Donaldson, 1996). This evidence was reported in the research literature twenty years ago (Liggins & Howie, 1972) as an unequivocal measure to reduce perinatal mortality and morbidity but until recently had not been comprehensively adopted. In Britain, the National Health Service in the late 1990s has placed research and development high on its list of priorities (Department of Health, 1995) and a great deal of attention has been given to the importance of ensuring that the benefits of research find their way into practice.

In the early 1990s, a new school of thought emerged which

sought to address, in a more fundamental and unified way, the need to promote more effective clinical practice. Evidence-based medicine has been described as a new paradigm for medical practice which seeks to reduce reliance on traditional factors such as intuition and unsystematic clinical experience and puts particular emphasis on the evaluation and use of evidence from clinical research (Evidence-Based Medicine Working Group, 1992). As these ideas have come to more widespread attention around the world, they have been greeted antagonistically by some sections of the medical profession. This is probably because they appear to cast aside traditional professional values based on judgement acquired through experience. Nevertheless, there has been a general acceptance of the need to move in this direction by many professional bodies and organisations as well as by health policy-makers. Indeed, enthusiasm for the concept has been such that it has broadened into notions of evidence-based health care, signifying the importance of bringing research knowledge to bear on decisions taken in the policy and management areas of health care, not purely the clinical.

It can be seen from Box 13.1 that the definition of evidence-based medicine suggests a fundamental change in the way that med-

Box 13.1   Definition of evidence-based practice

A process of life-long self-directed learning in which caring for one's own patients creates the need for clinically important information about diagnosis, prognosis, therapy, and other clinical and health care issues, and in which clinicians:

- convert these information needs into answerable questions;
- track down, with maximum efficiency, the best evidence with which to answer them (whether from clinical examination, the diagnostic laboratory, the published literature, or other sources);
- critically appraise that evidence for its validity (closeness to the truth) and usefulness (clinical applicability);
- apply the results of this appraisal in their clinical practice;
- evaluate their own performance.

Source: Sackett (1995)

icine is practised. Providing not just doctors but all health care professions with the means to scale these heights will require a realisation that the paradigm shift will not take place without support, leadership and an infrastructure of facilities. Thus, creating an environment in which an evidence-based approach becomes a routine part of everyday clinical practice for all health care professionals working within a health service is not a simple matter.

Achieving this change can seen as comprising three main steps. First, gathering, storing and making accessible research findings. Important in achieving this aim has been the process of supplementing traditional data bases of research literature (e.g. MEDLINE) with information in which whole fields of research have been reviewed, summarised and conclusions drawn. Prominent amongst these is the Cochrane Collaboration (Chalmers *et al.*, 1993) in which systematic reviews are conducted of randomised, controlled trials in particular fields of care and deposited in the data base for all to access. A systematic review is a form of secondary research. It takes the findings of primary research (the original studies) and evaluates them. Sometimes this will involve aggregating data from all the original studies and reanalysing them — a technique called meta-analysis. Although a systematic review is generally preferable to a single original study in determining the basis for clinical decisions, it is important to recognise that secondary research can also be good or bad and subject to bias. Thus, there are rules for conducting a high-quality systematic review (Deeks *et al.*, 1996) and there are traps for the unwary in relying on the results of meta-analysis (Thompson & Pocock, 1991).

The second step in achieving improvement in clinical practice involves assessing and making judgements about the evidence and formulating the changes to practice. Expertise is required in this process and so attention is increasingly being given to ensuring that health care professionals have training in so-called critical appraisal skills so that they have the ability to assess the validity and applicability of published research evidence to their practice (Bennett *et al.*, 1987). Beyond this, there is a need for expertise in, and understanding of, the process through which statements of clinical policy are produced. Formulating such statements — variously called 'clinical guidelines', 'clinical practice guidelines', 'clinical protocols', 'evidence-based recommendations' — is itself something which has been evaluated. Clinical practice guidelines have been used in a wide variety of clinical fields (Browman *et al.*, 1995). Systematic reviews of the evidence on the process of guideline formulation and its effectiveness have concluded that guidelines are more likely to be effective if: they are based upon evidence, they take into account local circumstances, they are disseminated by an active educational intervention and they incorporate patient specific reminders into the implementation process (Effective Health Care, 1994).

The third step in effecting a change towards evidence-based medicine involves strategies to ensure that practice actually changes. A major part of this process is making available the conclusions of reviews of evidence and promulgating clinical practice guidelines in a way which is tailored to the needs of decision-takers. Thus, there has been a growth in the number of publications which summarise the implications of research in user friendly form. Examples include the American College of Physicians (ACP) Journal Club; the Journal of Evidence-Based Medicine and various effectiveness bulletins (National Health Service Executive, 1996). Increasingly, such information is also available on the Internet (Kiley, 1996).

Despite such strategies, there is no guarantee that they will uniformly result in the uptake into clinical practice of research evidence. This is because it requires behaviour change on the part of health care professionals. Box 13.2 shows that a wide range of techniques have been demonstrated to be relevant in achieving such behaviour change. Donaldson (1996) has drawn attention to the

Box 13.2   Interventions that have been used to improve the performance of health care professionals and evaluated by trials

- Educational materials;
- Conferences;
- Outreach visits;
- Local opinion leaders;
- Patient-mediated interventions;
- Audit and feedback;
- Reminders;
- Marketing;
- Multifaceted interventions;
- Local consensus processes.

Source: Oxman (1994).

importance of evidence from the field of diffusion-utilisation research largely not concerned with health care but with applied psychology and communications theory. This work (Rogers 1995) shows that adoption of 'innovations' is a complex process involving the qualities of the innovation (or new behaviour) itself, the communication channels employed, the period of time and the social system concerned. Adoption is affected by factors such as: the perceived attributes of the change in question (e.g. observability, consistency with existing beliefs), whether communication is by mass media or face-to-face and the social structures of the organisation (particularly opinion leadership and networks). The importance of continuing professional education is also fundamental to the process of influencing the behaviour of practitioners. This has been an under-researched field but has more recently been the subject of effectiveness review (Davis et al., 1992).

Organisation-wide Measures

Mechanisms to improve quality which address the health care organisation as a whole have become more prominent with the emergence of health service management. The growth of managerialism in health services can be seen as due to five main influences (Donaldson, 1996): the need for cost containment; perceived benefits of bringing modern management strategies from other sectors into the health care environment; greater accountability to funding bodies for performance; the need to manage the processes and transactions of the health system; and, the introduction of a lay, in addition to a professional, view of service delivery.

As health care management has become a discipline in its own right, managers have sought to become properly equipped to do the job. Training programmes for modern health care managers will bring them into contact with theory and practice from other fields of management. Thus, issues such as leadership, organisational structure, quality management strategies have come to the fore in thinking about achieving quality goals because it is argued that they have been successful in other spheres of management.

Many of the popular approaches which have held sway in schools of management around the world might be described as 'guru-driven' with inspirational texts produced by thinkers like Charles Handy (Handy, 1985) and Tom Peters (Peters & Waterman, 1982) pointing to new directions for the leadership, culture, and structure of organisations. It could be argued that enthusiasm for such approaches have led to a tendency in health care organisations for restructuring, at times, for the sake of it. Nevertheless, it must always be remembered that a big part of the role of health care management lies in creating an organisational environment in which health care professionals can perform optimally. The effective health care manager will do this, for example, by creating the right culture, by communicating effectively, by providing information support, by aligning individual and organisational goals and by facilitating education and training (Donaldson, 1996).

In the future, it is likely that health care quality improvement philosophies will become aligned much more closely with the principles of total quality management and continuous quality improvement which are in place in other sectors and in which the leadership of organisations is a key to successful delivery. In this context, Deming's principles shown in Box 13.3 still offer a powerful challenge to those leading and managing health care organisations and many would probably admit that they fall far short of these ideals.

Accreditation, although not widely used in the United Kingdom, is another organisational quality improvement method with a long history of use in the United States, Canada and Australia. Scrivens (1995) observed that developments in the United Kingdom have tended to be small scale with the exception of the King's Fund Organisational Audit. She concluded that the process of applying for and achieving accreditation had beneficial effects on quality but noted that until there were additional rewards for participation and a clear policy position from government it was unlikely that widescale implementation would occur.

One of the most important examples of structured organisational quality review, although not strictly speaking accreditation, is the Malcolm Baldridge Award. Run by the United States Commerce Department the purpose of the Malcolm Baldridge Quality Award is to promote quality awareness, to recognise the quality achievements of United States companies and to publicise successful quality strategies. The awards cover manufacturing companies, service companies and small businesses. Applicants submit themselves to review on seven criteria: leadership, information and analysis, planning, human resource utilisation, quality assurance of products and services; quality results and customer satisfaction (National Institute of Standards and Technology, 1991). A rigorous process of examination and site visits precedes the awards which lay particular emphasis on the achievement of quality improvement.

Box 13.3 Deming's 14 obligations for management

1. Create constancy of purpose for continual improvement of products and service.
2. Adopt the new philosophy. We are now in a new economic age, created in Japan.
3. Eliminate the need for mass inspection as a way to achieve quality.
4. End the practice of awarding business solely on the basis of price tag.
5. Improve constantly and forever every process for planning, production and service.
6. Institute modern methods of training on the job.
7. Adopt and institute leadership aimed at helping people to do a better job.
8. Encourage effective two-way communication and other means to drive out fear throughout the organisation.
9. Break down barriers between departments and staff areas.
10. Eliminate the use of slogans, posters and exhortations.
11. Eliminate work standards that prescribe numerical quotas for the workforce and numerical goals for people in management.
12. Remove the barriers that rob hourly workers, and people in management, of their right to pride of workmanship.
13. Institute a vigorous programme of education, and encourage self-improvement for everyone.
14. Clearly define top management's permanent commitment to ever-improving quality and productivity.

Source: Deming (1986).

There are other methods through which external review and validation of a health care organisation's work can serve to improve quality by enabling action to be taken to meet targets set or implement recommendations made. These include reviews by independent external agencies (e.g. in England, the Audit Commission and the National Audit Office); voluntary schemes for fulfilling criteria for quality recognition (e.g. in Britain, the British Standards Institute's BS 5750 award); regulatory or quasi-regulatory bodies (e.g. in the United States, the Joint Commission on Accreditation of

Health Care Organisations, JCAHO; in England, the Clinical
Standards Advisory Group, CSAG).

The Empowerment of Patients

In recent years, the importance of patients in strategies for quality
improvement has been recognised. However, patients are likely to
make judgements about quality based on a whole range of information some of which is not recognised in mainstream thinking about
health care quality. For example, personal experience and word of
mouth and reading media reports could be more important than
informing themselves using patient information leaflets and databases or by seeking specific advice from experts. Changing this so
that the patient really has a role in quality improvement requires an
actively managed strategy.

Traditionally, ensuring that there is a patient's perspective in
quality improvement has involved the operation of a complaints
procedure. Complaints made by patients about their care do represent an important way for lessons to be learned about lapses in quality of care which can then be translated into quality improvements.
Patients will wish to see their concerns taken seriously, their com-
plaint investigated, a clear explanation given and follow-up action
taken (Donaldson & Cavanagh, 1992). Whilst an important element
in judging the quality of a health service will be how effectively
complaints are dealt with, patient participation in quality improvement must go beyond a good complaints system.

Seeking patients' views on services proactively rather than relying on complaints has grown in importance in recent years but
some of the methodological issues are quite complex. Macintyre &
Kleman (1994) suggest that the approaches available can be cate-
gorised in three levels which reflect a movement from a reactive to
a proactive and dynamic approach to patient involvement. Level
one is characterised by a reactive stance where organisations do not
seek to understand the consumers' perspective. Complaints are the
typical method of data collection with little or no trend analysis. In
such a scenario lessons are not learned and the approach is event
based. Level two is where the organisation seeks actively to listen to
customers. A variety of channels are opened up and active feedback
is sought. Regular unstructured consumer surveys, telephone hot
lines or help desks are examples of the type of approach used to
gather data and to provide feedback. Trends are identified and
action is taken to remedy shortcomings. Level three requires organ-

isations to search for and understand customers' expectation. A systems-wide approach is taken and the lessons learned in one department are considered for relevance to other parts of the organisation. Specially designed surveys that get behind superficial responses, focus groups that explore issues in detail and customer interviews that result in data that then impart meaning and understanding of the customer's perspective are used.

In the National Health Service in Britain, 'The Patients Charter' (Secretary of State for Health, 1991) has produced and published rights and standards which patients should expect from local services. Giving the public comparative information on the outcome of care in different services is also seen by some as important because it releases the additional force of consumer pressure to achieve beneficial change. This approach has been more widely used in the United States, than in Britain, where it is often termed the 'report card' and applied to fields such as mortality from coronary heart disease treatment. Despite the fact that the proposed reforms of the United States health care system did not go ahead as set out in the President Clinton's Health Security Plan, increased amounts of data on health service quality have become available via HEDIS reporting (Health Plan Employer Data and Information Set — the Health Maintenance Organisation report card).

One of the main problems with this kind of information is that it usually provokes sensationalist media reporting which tends to produce a defensive reaction on the part of the health care organisations which are perceived as poor performers. Creation of this kind of blame culture is likely over time to lead to organisations being less open and honest about their performance. The hostility of physicians is often also aroused. Indeed, clinicians will often react by criticising the quality of the data (in many cases, with some justification). In the United States, longer experience with the routine public use of these measures suggests that perverse incentives will begin to operate. For example, in the interests of optimising performance, hospitals may make subtle changes to limit the access to high risk patients. It seems inevitable, though, that public disclosure of information on service quality will become more common in the future and the difficulties inherent in this process will have to be overcome.

MEASUREMENT

Measuring the quality of care provided is also a complex field. The issues have been addressed in studies, by developmental work in individual health care organisations and by inspectorial, standard setting, regulatory and professional bodies. Most attention has been given to developing measures within specific fields of quality assessment, particularly outcome and process measures. In the British National Health Service, the measures of quality of care in routine use have serious limitations. Indicators such as response time, length of hospital stay, unadjusted hospital case fatality rates, numbers of complaints made are available and are used in managing the service. However, they provide poor insights into the quality of care provided. In addition, because of the difficulty in developing robust, sensitive and reliable measures of quality there has been a tendency to over-specify standards which focus on input or throughput. Popper (1992) has noted that such approaches result in considerable resources being expended on data capture thereby diverting effort from direct care delivery, hence potentially adversely affecting quality.

Quality data based upon outcomes traditionally have reflected the endpoints of illness and the health experience. Lohr (1988) has referred to these as the five 'Ds': death, disease, disability, discomfort and dissatisfaction. Much of the development of detailed outcome measures has occurred within particular areas of specialist medical practice or in particular chronic disease populations. For example Cope et al. (1987) reported studies examining the success rates for cardiac arrest procedures for individual hospital departments. Shaw (1989) provided a detailed critique of the limitations of such approaches highlighting the difficulties of collecting comparable outcome data particularly if clinical staff were not committed to, and involved in, the process. Perhaps the most consistent concern raised regarding the use of condition-specific outcome indicators has been the need to ensure that measures are adjusted for severity and co-existing pathology. There are obvious methodological problems in making comparisons on the relative performance of health services using outcome data. Any variation may be explained by the characteristics of patients (age, disease severity), by the size of the patient populations being compared, or by the presence of other factors which affect outcome but which do not form part of the assessment or analysis. There are examples of practical applications which have addressed these problems and sought to provide severity adjusted outcome measures (Pine & Harper, 1994).

Other outcome measures include those focusing on: quality of life; functional status or activities of daily living, health status; family or carer stress; patient satisfaction. However, it is often difficult to access the measures used in such studies and difficult to obtain information on the reliability and validity of the scales used. To this end, a number of authors have endeavoured to collect and publish such information (McDowell & Newell, 1987; Waltz & Strickland, 1988).

Another approach to the measurement of quality is the application of a tracer methodology. Kessner *et al.* (1973) advocate that, for assessing the quality of a health care system, tracers are needed which are discrete, identifiable health problems. It is argued that the manner in which they are addressed will illuminate how the system as a whole is performing.

In health care, measurement of quality can be based on the process aspects of care in examining the care provided against criteria of best practice. The issues in this field have been reviewed by Irvine & Donaldson (1993). Assessment of the performance of processes of service are part of the philosophy of total quality management. The aim of statistical process control, well described in the work of Deming (1986), seeks to measure the quality of the process by exploring the extent and source of variation in the operation of a system. Correcting these problems is seen as a particularly effective way of improving the quality of the service — perhaps summed up in the aphorism: 'fix the system not the problem'.

A particularly imaginative conceptualisation of the aims of a comprehensive system to assess quality in health care is shown in Box 13.4. Unfortunately few health care organisations can yet claim to meet all such criteria. There remains scope for improvement as well as considerable need for further research to assess health care quality in a way which will explore all the perspectives raised in this chapter.

CONCLUSIONS

Over the last three decades, there has been major progress in developing new concepts and philosophies to explore the meaning of quality in health care. This has opened up many different perspectives which have, at times, seemed to diverge. It remains a stimulating and exciting field of health services research and practice in which public health has an important role to play.

In the future, it will be important to draw together these different strands to ensure that strategies for quality improvement are integrated. It seems increasingly likely that this will occur at the level of the health care organisation. It is here that a culture can be

Box 13.4   Aims of a system to assess quality of health care

- decrease underuse and overuse;
- assess outcomes;
- based on the best possible synthesis of knowledge and judgement;
- puts explicit standards and criteria in the public domain, as is true of all other industries;
- involves public disclosure of results;
- has a conceptual model that ties deficiencies to preventive or corrective actions;
- accurate, valid, and reliable information is available for consumer choice;
- tools and information are available to improve quality.

Source: Brook (1994).

created, through excellence in leadership, in which professional and management-based quality improvement methods become part of an organisation-wide quality strategy (Fig.13.2). The public health perspective will continue to view the impact of this not just within local health care organisations but through the currency of population health need and overall health improvement.

REFERENCES

Bennett K J, Sackett D L, Haynes R B, Neufeld V R, Tugwell P, Roberts R 1987 A controlled trial of teaching critical appraisal of the clinical literature to medical students. Journal of the American Medical Association; 257: 2451–4

Berwick DM 1989 Continuous improvement as an ideal in health care. New England Journal of Medicine 320: 53–6

Blain P, Donaldson LJ 1995 The reporting of inpatient suicides: identifying the problem. Public Health 109: 293–301

Brook RH 1994 What will health care reform look like? Journal on Quality Improvement 20: 472–3

Browman GP Levine MN, Mohide EA, Hayward RSA, Pritchard KI, Gafni A, Laupacis A. 1995 The practice guidelines development cycle: a conceptual tool for practice guidelines development and implementation. Journal of Clinical Oncology 13: 502–12

Chalmers I, Enkin M, Keirse MJ 1993 Preparing and updating systematic reviews of randomised controlled trials of health care. Milbank Quarterly 71: 411–37.

Charlton JRH, Hartley RM, Silver R, Holland WW 1983 Geographical variation in mortality from conditions amenable to medical intervention in England and Wales. Lancet i: 691–6

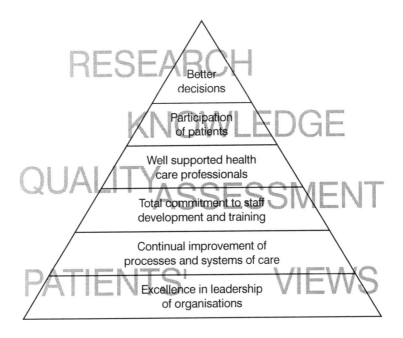

Fig. 13.2   Building successful quality improvement in health care.

Codman EA 1914 The product of a hospital. Surgery, Gynaecology and Obstetrics 18: 491–6

Cope AR, Quinton DN, Dove AF, Sloan JP, Dave SH 1987 Survival from cardiac arrest in the emergency department. Journal of the Royal Society of Medicine 80: 746–9

Davis DA, Thomson MA, Oxman AD, Haynes RB 1992 Evidence for the effectiveness of CME: a review of 50 randomised controlled trials. Journal of the American Medical Association; 268: 1111–17

Deeks J, Glanville J, Sheldon T 1996 Undertaking systematic reviews of effectiveness: guidelines for those carrying out or commissioning reviews. CRD Publications, York

Deming WE 1986 Out of the crisis. Massachusetts Institute of Technology, Cambridge

Department of Health 1995 Research and development: towards an evidence-based health service. DoH, London

Donabedian A 1966 Evaluating the quality of medical care. Milbank Memorial Fund Quarterly 4: 166–206

Donabedian A 1989 Institutional and professional responsibilities in quality assurance. Quality Assurance in Health Care 1: 3–11

Donaldson LJ 1996 Impact of management on outcomes. In Scientific Basis of Health Services eds MP Peckham, R Smith. BMJ Publishing Group, London

Donaldson LJ, Cavanagh J 1992 Clinical complaints and their handling: a time for change. Quality in Health Care 1: 21–25

Donaldson RJ, Donaldson LJ 1993 Essential Public Health Medicine. Kluwer, London

Eddy DM 1982 Clinical policies and the quality of clinical practice. New England Journal of Medicine 307: 343–7

Effective Health Care 1994 Implementing clinical practice guidelines: can guidelines be used to improve clinical practice. University of Leeds

Evidence-based Medicine Working Group. Evidence-based medicine: a new approach to teaching the practice of medicine. Journal of American Medical Association 1992; 268: 2420–25

Handy C 1985 Understanding organisations, 3rd Edn. Penguin Books, London

Hopkins A 1993 What do we mean by appropriate health care? Report of a working group prepared for the Director of Research and Development. Quality in Health Care 2: 117–23

Irvine DH, Donaldson LJ 1993 Quality and standards in health care. Proceedings of the Royal Society of Edinburgh 101B: 1–30.

Joint Commission of Accreditation of Health Care Organisations (JCAHO) 1989 Quality assurance in managed health care organisations. JCAHO, Chicago

Kessner DM, Kalk CE, Singer J 1973 Assessing Health Quality—The Case For Tracers. New England Journal of Medicine 288: 189–94

Kiley R 1996 Medical Information on the Internet. Churchill Livingstone, London

Kitson AI, Hyndman SJ, Harvey G, Yerrell PH 1990 Quality Patient Care: The Dynamic Standard Setting System. Scutari, Harrow

Lembcke PA 1967 Evolution of the medical audit. Journal of the American Medical Association 199: 543–50

Liggins GC, Howie RN 1972 A controlled trial of antepartum glucocorticoid treatment for prevention of the respiratory distress syndrome in premature infants. Paediatrics 50: 515–25

Lilford RJ 1997 Hysterectomy: will it pay the bills in 2007? British Medical Journal 314: 160–1

Lohr KN 1988 Outcome measurement: concepts and questions. Inquiry 25: 37–50

Macintyre K, Kleman CC 1994 Measuring Customer Satisfaction In Continuous Quality Improvement in Health Care: Theory, Implementation and Applications. Eds CP Mclaughlin, AD Kaluzny; Aspen Publishers, Gaithersburg, Maryland

Maxwell R 1984 Quality assessment in health. British Medical Journal 288: 1470–2

McDowell I, Newell C 1987 Measuring Health: A guide to rating scales and questionnaires. Oxford University Press, Oxford

National Health Service Executive 1996 Clinical effectiveness: reference pack. NHSE, Leeds

National Institute of Standards and Technology 1991 Malcolm Baldridge National Quality Award — 1991 fact sheet. National Institute of Standards and Technology, Gaithersburg, Maryland

Oxman AD 1994 No magic bullets: a systematic review of 102 trials of interventions to help health care professionals deliver services more effectively and efficiently. North Thames Regional Health Authority, London

Peters T, Waterman RK 1982 In Search of Excellence. Harper & Row, New York

Pine M, Harper D 1994 Designing and using case mix indices. Managed Care Quarterly 2: 1–11

Popper C 1992 Studies in decentralisation and quasi-markets 9: Quasi-markets, contracts and quality. University of Bristol,

Rogers EM 1995 Diffusion of innovations. 4th edn. Free Press, New York

Rutstein DD, Berenberg W, Chalmers TC, Child CG, Fishman AP, Perrin EB. 1976. Measuring the quality of health care; a clinical method. New England Journal of Medicine 294: 582–8

Sackett D 1995 The Centre for Evidence-Based Medicine. Milton Keynes: Anglia and Oxford Regional Health Authority.

Scrivens E. 1995. Accreditation: Protecting The Professional Or The Consumer? Open University Press, Buckingam

Secretary of State for Health 1991 The Patient's Charter: Raising the standard. HMSO, London

Secretary of State For Health 1996. The National Health Service: A Service With Ambitions. Cm 3425. The Stationery Office, London

Shaw CD 1989 Clinical outcome indicators. Health Trends 21: 37–40

Thompson SG, Pocock SJ 1991 Can meta-analyses be trusted? Lancet 338: 1127–30

Waltz CF, Strickland OL 1988 Measurement of Nursing Outcomes: Volume One Measuring Client Outcomes. Springer, New York

World Health Organisation Working Group 1989 The principles of quality assurance. Quality Assurance in Health Care 1: 79–95

14. Public Health and Ethics

Robin Downie and Jane Macnaughton

INTRODUCTION

From the time of Hippocrates until the 1960s medical ethics (or health care ethics or bio-ethics) were seen in terms of doctors' duties to patients. These duties have traditionally been thought of as those of not harming the patient (non-maleficence) and of helping the patient (beneficence). Codes of medical ethics and philosophical discussion from the 1970s increasingly added 'respect for patient's autonomous decisions' to the duties of non-maleficence and beneficence.

Now, whereas medical ethics based on non-maleficence and beneficence can easily be extended to cover many public health interventions, which are intended to be 'for our own good', there are greater problems for public health ethics if autonomy is made a central concept. To bring this out, we shall contrast the interventions typical of clinical medicine with those of public health medicine. It should be noted here that we are using in this chapter the definition of public health accepted by the UK in the Acheson Report (1988):

Public health is the science and art of preventing disease, prolonging life and promoting health through organised efforts of society.

Assuming this definition we can contrast the approach of clinical medicine with that of public health medicine.

HEALTH CARE ETHICS AND PUBLIC HEALTH ETHICS

The clinician is typically in a one-to-one relationship with a patient who has requested an interview because of a felt problem. The clinical imperative is therefore that something must be done including the giving of advice. The public health specialist, on the other hand, does not have a specific patient with whom he is in a special relationship, and has received no request from a patient. It could be said that the public health specialist responds to a collective cry from individuals in a community when some medical problem occurs which affects a large number of people in a locality. One recent example is the outbreak of *Eschericia coli* 0157 in Wishaw in central Scotland in 1996. But here, again, there is no continuing relationship between the specialist and the affected group of individuals and therefore no opportunity for those individuals to express their views on the public health response. The public health specialist therefore is (a) making a judgement about what it is in people's interest to have, whether they have requested it or not, and (b) dealing with populations, groups or societies rather than individuals. The ethical consequence of these features are that public health generates problems concerned with issues such as paternalism and individual rights, which are broadly (i.e. non-party) political in their implications. It follows that for any specific intervention (legislation for clean water, a programme of immunisation, restriction on smoking in public places or whatever), the necessary precondition of implementation is that it will improve the health of the public — and this improvement must be objectively demonstrable (Charlton 1993). According to this approach, effectiveness must be established by scientific means, such that all rational and competent judges can agree on the facts (Kelly & Charlton 1992). The most common technique for establishing effectiveness of this kind is through the discipline of epidemiology, in which clear and certain conclusions may not always be obtainable. The importance of having measurable objectives for programme management and evaluation has been recognised in some official documents. See, for example, the Surgeon General's Report, *Healthy People 2000* (1991), or, in England, the Report of the Department of Health, *The Health of the Nation* (1992), or Tones and Tilfors (1994).

JUSTICE AND UTILITY IN PUBLIC HEALTH MEDICINE

It follows from above that public interventions will require to be supported by two further ethical principles: justice and utility. In this section we shall examine a number of contexts in which these principles create the ethical framework for public health policies. But first let us examine the principles.

Justice and Utility: the Principles

Justice sometimes means treating individual patients justly, say, by observing their rights, and sometimes that autonomous patients are all equally entitled to shares in the distribution of health care. The latter emphasis is particularly important for public health. Indeed, it is arguable that justice (or equity) raises the most important of the ethical issues for public health. There are variable levels of health between countries, and within countries there are marked differences in health which can be correlated with differences in distribution of resources (Whitehead, 1987).

In discussions of justice it is important to distinguish 'equity' and 'equality'. The distinction can best be described by looking at those factors which can influence health and health care. It is possible to divide inequalities into those which are unavoidable, and hence where questions of equity do not arise, and those which might be avoided and thus raise issues of equity. Let us look at some examples (Whitehead, 1990). In discussing the examples, we must always remember that what is 'unavoidable' at one point in history becomes 'avoidable' at another.

First, natural or biological variations such as age, sex, and race and genetic background could be considered as factors which cannot be changed and thus any inequalities related to them are unavoidable. For example, older men have a higher incidence of heart disease than younger men, a clear example of an inequality. But no one would consider this related to inequity, except to the extent that we have neglected risk factor reduction in the elderly (Omenn 1990; Hermanson et al., 1988).

Secondly, lifestyle and behaviour, if freely chosen, can result in inequalities in health. As an example, cigarette smokers have a higher incidence of lung cancer than non-smokers. This is an inequality, but to the extent that it is created by choice, it is not inequitable. Indeed, selective uptake of health promotional initiatives, for example, by middle class groups, could even increase inequalities in health, but could not be considered as unfair, unless it could be established that health promotion is selectively targeted on these groups.

Thirdly, lifestyle and behaviour, if not freely chosen, and which results in poor health, is likely to be considered as avoidable by society and thus unfair. A behaviour chosen through a lack of resources, housing conditions, overcrowding, dangerous working conditions, exposure to environmental hazards, or lack of adequate public health response, would be an example of this. Disabled people often suffer unfairness (inequity) which compounds their already unequal health.

Fourthly, inadequate access to health care or other public services might be inequitable if the cause were avoidable. For example, financial considerations which resulted in a failure to use transport might be one such factor. Another might be lack of access to information about services due to learning or language problems, or the information not being available. This lack, or inequity, could lead to inequalities of access because of the restriction of choice and opportunity.

In summary of this discussion of the principle of justice, we can say that those examples bring out that equity is about fairness and justice and implies that everyone should have an opportunity to attain his or her full potential for health. Inequalities exist in health and health care. Some of these are unavoidable, and thus could not be considered unfair or inequitable. Others are avoidable. It is this latter group in which the inequalities are inequitable, to which further attention might be addressed.

In discussion of public health we must also stress the principle of utility — of maximising the benefits for the populations involved. Utility is the principle concerned with the maximising of outcomes or preferences. In the old formulation it tells us to seek the greatest happiness of the greatest number. As such the principle of utility says nothing about how the greatest happiness should be distributed: an aggregate of utility A might be greater than an aggregate of B, but we might still give our moral approval to the situation which produces B rather than A, on the grounds that in B the benefits are more fairly distributed. Thus, there must be a balance between the ethical forces of justice and of utility.

Justice and Utility: Prioritising

Some people may argue that prioritising or rationing, while it raises important policy issues, does not raise ethical issues. The assumption of this position is that ethics has to do only with the face-to-face situation. We believe this view to be inadequate. Questions of the supply and fair distribution of resources are matters of ethics, and the general ethical principles which are relevant are those of utility and justice. Ethical problems of prioritising arise in the area of health service provision. The level of provision of health services is of considerable importance particularly in relation to the balance between hospital and primary care, the use of resources to develop effective interventions, and the ability to deliver public health measures. The infrastructural organisation and management are all important.

In recent years in Britain the government has been laying emphasis on Primary Care as the central plank of the National

Health Service with talk of a 'primary care-led health service' (Bogle & Chisholm, 1996). This approach has clear advantages for a publicly funded service in that the care provided by general practitioners is much cheaper than hospital care and it makes sense to provide as much care for patients locally near their own homes by doctors whom they know and who know them.

One of the ways in which the government has attempted to promote the power of general practice within the health service is by the creation of fundholding practices. Fund holders can negotiate for services from a range of local hospitals and can choose where to buy services for their patients based on the quality of care provided and the price. For the first time this has given GPs real muscle in influencing the development and scope of services provided by hospitals. The idea is that GPs know their patients and know what services they need; therefore, as the slogan goes, 'the money follows the patient'.

This move has, however, created the possibility of an unequal share of primary care resources going to fundholding practices at the expense of non-fundholders as fundholding (with its need for extra management staff to negotiate contracts) is more expensive than conventional general practice (Stewart-Brown et al., 1996) and concern has been expressed about the creation of a 'two tier' service (Kammerling & Kinnear, 1996). The problem is that the primary care resource cake is no bigger than it was: it is just being cut up differently and, inevitably, some GPs and their patients will get a smaller slice.

Within primary care there is, therefore, a debate about the allocation of resources, but, since the change of emphasis to a 'primary care-led health service' there has been an increasing transfer of work from secondary to primary care (Roland, 1996) and funding has not followed this transfer. This has led to a vigorous debate about the allocation of resources between primary and secondary care. The NHS in Britain works on the basis that each person must come through their GP to get access to expensive secondary care resources. The assumption is that GPs are aware of the limited nature of these resources and will refer wisely and equitably. The government and health service planners recognise the crucial position of GPs as gatekeepers of NHS resources and are attempting to redress the balance of power through past and future (Department of Health, 1996) proposals to improve the status of general practice within the NHS. If funding does not follow this shift of emphasis however, these moves could destabilise the structure of the NHS.

Justice and Utility: Prevention

There is sometimes confusion between prevention, which is the abolition or reduction in the incidence of the disease; avoidance, which is keeping clear of risk factors; and protection, which may limit the spread of disease, say by vaccination or immunisation. For example, public health policy may encourage the prevention of malaria by swamp-clearing programmes and thus aim at the elimination of the source of the disease; or travellers may be prevented from catching the disease by avoiding certain geographical areas; or they may be protected against it by being given tablets. All these practices are loosely called 'prevention'. Of course, the categories will sometimes overlap. For instances, immunisation or vaccination programmes, which are really protection programmes, may lead to a reduction in the incidence of a disease, or even to its elimination, as in the case of smallpox. But this overlap does not always occur. The compulsory wearing of seatbelts is often regarded as a preventive measure. But it does not prevent accidents; only good driving and safer roads and vehicles do that. It gives a measure of protection against accidents (Blaney, 1987).

It might seem that there is no need to provide any ethical justification for prevention: it is self-evidently a good thing. While this may be true, the general public and governments do not always act as if it were so. From the point of view of government, it seems that much more money goes in the direction of health care than of prevention, and from the point of view of the public there is often an attitude of scepticism towards many preventive measures, and even more towards what is now called 'health promotion'. Prevention as a general policy therefore requires some justification. There is an economical justification, that prevention is usually cheaper than care; medical justification, that some diseases are probably not completely curable so their occurrence should be prevented: and an ethical justification, that prevention avoids the pain, misery and grief of disease. It is also possible to include the economic and medical justifications in a wide sense of 'ethical justification'. As we shall see, however, this general ethical justification of prevention does not always apply to specific areas of prevention, and even when it does there are those who argue that the benefits of prevention can be outweighed in some cases by the ethical costs. Let us look at some examples.

Take the fluoridation of local water supplies. From the 1930s it was noted that there was a correlation between levels of fluoride in the drinking water and levels of dental caries. This suggested a preventive policy of introducing fluoride where the level was low.

There were objections, on the grounds of undesirable side-effects, such as Down's Syndrome and more recently cancer. But a Working Party in Britain (1985) found no evidence for such claims, and other scientific groups have reached the same conclusion. The ethical objection remains, however, that adding fluoride to the water supply can count as compulsory medication, and as such it is a violation of individual rights as laid down in the UN Declaration of Human Rights. Rights, of course, are not inalienable and can be overridden when the survival of the public requires it. But it is doubtful if the prevention of dental caries can count as a justification for ignoring rights. Note that there is really no solution to this dispute. One position or the other must be overruled (Knox, 1987).

The issue of vaccination for rubella raises rather different issues. The vaccine for rubella works by providing a benefit to the children of those to whom it is given. Now the vaccine can be given to girls only or to both girls and boys. If it is given to girls only, there is little effect on the transmission or eradication of the disease. A 'girls only' policy is therefore a 'protection' rather than a 'prevention' measure. If, on the other hand, the vaccine is given to both girls and boys, and if the uptake is over 90%, we have a preventive measure which will eventually lead to the eradication of the disease. But, if the second policy is followed and the uptake is low, say about 60%, then we have a situation which is harmful to the children of the unvaccinated young female population, for they will be much less likely to develop natural immunity. The ethical issues, then, are these. If we (the public) want the benefits of prevention then we must also put up with a degree of compulsion to ensure a high uptake. If compulsion is ethically or politically unacceptable, then the best policy, to avoid harm, is to offer protection to those at risk. Again, there is no ethically correct answer; a choice must be made (Knox, 1987).

Justice and Utility: Screening

Another public health activity which falls in general terms into the category of prevention is that of screening. Screening can be defined in various ways, but a simple definition is provided by Stone and Stewart (1994): 'Screening is a preventive activity which seeks to identify an unsuspected disease or pre-disease condition for which an effective intervention is available'. Screening is currently a fashionable medical activity. The demand for it is being encouraged by governments and by certain patients' organisations.

Politically, it seems desirable because there is a belief that prevention saves money, and successive governments have therefore set up various screening programmes. A national screening programme for cervical cancer was set up in the UK in 1964, and a programme for breast cancer was established in 1988 for women aged 50–64 years. The establishment of such programmes has been enthusiastically supported by various women's groups. Indeed, such is the current demand for screening that Shickle and Chadwick (1994) in a discussion of the ethics of screening ask whether 'screeningitis' is an incurable disease. If it were, no doubt there would be demand for a screening programme!

It is possible to screen for many conditions, but screening programmes must satisfy ethical criteria. First, they must satisfy the informed consent criterion for any sort of medical intervention. Secondly, since screening initiatives tend to be profession driven rather than individual driven, there is an additional responsibility for the professional to justify the intervention which may not have been requested. Thirdly, some screening procedures carry health risks, and all of them are likely to be accompanied by discomfort, anxiety, and inconvenience for symptomless individuals. Fourthly, any screening programme carries with it the risks of the false-positive or the false-negative. Thus screening requires as much ethical justification as other medical interventions. Moreover, since screening programmes can be expensive in the aggregate, they require evaluation. Once again, therefore, the ethical principles of justice and utility must be used in the justification of screening programmes.

Ethical Problems of Health Promotion: Health

The Acheson Report definition of public health makes it clear that public health medicine must not only prevent disease but promote health. The literature of the new public health, and especially health promotion, tends nowadays to have a complex view of the concept of health and to distinguish various elements within it.

The first of those is often called 'negative health', or the absence of ill-health. Ill-health itself is a complex notion comprising disease, illness, handicap, injury and other related ideas. These overlapping concepts can be linked if they are seen on the model of abnormal, unwanted or incapacitating states of a biological system.

The second idea of 'positive health' has appeared more recently in published reports. The origins of this idea are in the definition of health to be found in the preamble to the Constitution of the WHO.

Health is a state of complete physical, mental and social well-being, and not merely the absence of disease or infirmity (WHO, 1946)

It follows from this definition that 'well-being' is an important ingredient in positive health.

A third idea in the concept of health is that of 'fitness'. Fitness in its most obvious sense refers to the state of someone's heart and lungs. To be fit in this sense is to have a place on a scale ranging from being able to climb stairs or run for a bus without getting out of breath to being able to run a marathon or climb Mount Everest. Fitness can also be used in a related but broader sense, which we might call 'sociological' as opposed to the 'heart and lungs' sense. In the sociological sense of fitness a person is fit *for* some occupation or job. This means that people have the necessary health to enable them to perform the job or task adequately without, for example, too many days off work.

The WHO definition refers to the 'mental and social' as well as to the physical. Nevertheless, the mental and social components of health are the poor relations of the health services and do not receive adequate attention. It is certainly true that mental health is most often taken to be the absence of mental ill-health. The idea of positive mental health or mental well-being is an obscure one, and perhaps it is ethically dangerous if it implies that eccentricity and single-mindedness are to be discouraged and the balanced and conformist personality encouraged.

The idea of 'social well-being' is, in fact, just as obscure as that of mental well-being, although at first sight it does not seem to be a difficult notion. What does it mean? In one sense 'social well-being' refers to the skills and other abilities which enable us to form friendships and relate to other people in conversation and through the many different sorts of contact which are part of ordinary social life. Sometimes these are called 'lifeskills', and the possession of them helps to create a sense of 'self-esteem' which is currently a fashionable concept in the literature of health education. Clearly, like fitness, social well-being in this sense can be graded on a scale from negative to positive. It is a property of individuals and refers to their ability to cope in a social context — hence 'social well-being' is an appropriate term.

Can we link the absence of ill-health and the presence of well-being in a single concept of health in the manner of the WHO definition? This is not a rarefied question because it affects the legitimate scope of health education. If well-being is a component in the concept of health, then clearly health education has a much wider remit than it would otherwise have.

One important factor influencing this question is that ill-health and well-being cannot be related to each other as opposite poles on a linear scale. This approach has been tried by some theorists but it is not satisfactory, for it is logically possible (and not in fact uncommon) for someone to have poor physical health but a high state of well-being — as in the case of a terminal patient in a hospice who is supported by caring staff and loving friends — or a good state of physical health but poor well-being — as in the case of someone who has no diseases or illnesses but lacks friends, a job, interests.

The fact that health (the absence of ill-health) and well-being cannot be related on a linear scale must raise the question of whether they are in fact two components of a single concept. It can be argued that they are aspects of a single concept (Downie, Tannahill, Tannahill, 1996). But it may be preferable and less confusing conceptually to think of them as two overlapping concepts rather than as a single concept with two dimensions. Thus the feeling of well-being that a person has after an invigorating swim can fairly be described as a 'glow of health', but the well-being or satisfaction that a person has after writing a chapter in a book, listening to a piece of music, or just playing an enjoyable game is less obviously related to concepts of health, and more obviously related to concepts such as 'enjoyment' and 'happiness'. Again, the well-being that is created by moving someone to better housing is more obviously related to concepts of 'welfare' than to that of health. Our conclusion is that, while the concepts of health and well-being overlap, they are distinct and cannot be combined into one concept.

But whether we think of health as a single multi-faceted concept, or as a narrower concept which overlaps with related concepts such as well-being and fitness, we must still examine two charges sometimes levelled at health promotional activities — that they are unethical in that they are 'imperialistic', and 'commercialise' health.

Health Promotion: Imperialism

Those making the charge of health imperialism might argue that what in health promotion terms is 'positive health' is really just a name for a range of states which are as easily or better seen in other ways. For example, 'well-being' is just another name for happiness. Again, the idea of 'fitness' might be said to be a technical one, relative to specific ends, such as playing in the Premier League, but not one with an important bearing on health. Mental illness may satisfy some of the criteria for illness (although even that has been disputed), but positive mental health might be said by critics to be a concept which attempts to annex the territory of the well adjusted to that of the healthy. For example, mental illnesses, such as depressions or obsessions, are incapacitating in a manner similar to that of physical illness, but to stress positive mental health might be seen as simply making a value judgement in favour of the conventional or the well balanced as opposed to the eccentric, as we have already noted.

In reply to this sort of objection, it is helpful to introduce the concept of health alliances. There are certain activities which are indisputably health promotion, but there are many others with which health promotion can form alliances. If health and health promotion can be seen in this logically and practically flexible way, then the charge of imperialism can be avoided.

Health Promotion: Commercialism

The second ethical objection to health promotion is that it attempts to bypass autonomy and to sell health like a commodity. In this it might be said to resemble the advertisements for unhealthy products which it is opposing (Williams, 1984).

In reply to this argument we might question the premise that autonomy is something which everyone in fact possesses. People can be victims of all sorts of social processes and be lacking in power. For example, as the advertising of tobacco and alcohol becomes progressively more difficult in some countries, so the manufacturers have turned their attention to the developing world, and the huge markets which are opening up. As the countries become more affluent, so the consumption of such products increase with consequential long-term adverse health effects. Another example concerns breast milk substitutes. All health authorities are clear about the value of breast feeding for the mother and the baby. However, considerable pressure was brought to bear on mothers in developing countries to use breast milk substitutes. Not only would this be more expensive, but the health benefits of breast feeding would be lost. International action was required to deal with this issue. The WHO resolved that states ensure that there be no free or subsidised substitute, which would affect breast feeding practice. This may seem to be merely a political compromise, but it may nevertheless be an effective way of implementing an ethically defensible position.

In view of the political and commercial power of the anti-health forces in society, health must be presented in as attractive a way as possible or health education will fail totally. If health educators confine themselves strictly to the rational, critical approach to education, then it is preferable to depict health education as an element within a larger health promotion movement concerned with health advocacy, legislative change, fiscal reform, and the mobilisation of community interests, as well as education narrowly conceived.

The tension between the ethical requirement to be person-respecting in methods and the practical necessity to be effective is addressed from an interesting point of view in the literature of self-help groups. The growth of self-care groups concerned with every conceivable malady and involving both the sufferers and their relatives has been a notable development during the last decade. These movements avoid the charge of paternalism commonly still made against every branch of health care, including health education. Apart from ethical considerations, self-care movements seem to be effective within their limits, although they may benefit from a professional health educator to advise and facilitate. Advising and facilitating is indeed an important role for health education.

PUBLIC HEALTH AND 'THE ORGANISED EFFORTS OF SOCIETY'

Public health medicine, according to the Acheson Report definition, must obtain its results 'through the organised efforts of society'. How are we to interpret this, and what ethical issues arise from our interpretation? Is it just a metaphor to speak of 'society' bringing about health? One obvious answer to this question is that to speak of 'society' bringing about health is a roundabout way of referring to our elected political representatives. We shall therefore begin by looking at the role of the state in health care, concentrating on health legislation.

Legislation and Prevention

First, a person's right to exercise autonomy may be legitimately curtailed by health legislation when he or she is suffering from certain sorts of infectious disease or mental illness such that the interests or health of others are liable to be harmed. There is no difficulty about the acceptance of this restriction in general terms. The problems arise over the more detailed application. For example, a topical question concerns the nature and extent of the restrictions which should be placed on sufferers from AIDS, or the extent of justifiable investigations or reporting of those who may be HIV-positive (Walters, 1988). Again, it is controversial how far those who are mentally ill should be detained against their will, or what sort of treatment they should have if they are detained.

Pressure for legislation is generated as more becomes known about how diseases are transmitted. For example, the dangers of 'passive smoking' are now appreciated, and other sorts of environmental pollution are now known to cause or exacerbate diseases such as asthma. There is therefore a case for curbing the freedom of both individuals and corporate bodies, such as industries, in the name of the autonomy of other individuals. This issue is, of course, a source of much political debate. Some countries have banned smoking in many public places, and various 'watch-dogs' keep a close eye on the consequences of the operation of the nuclear power industry. Although there can be political debate about applications of the 'preventing harm to others' idea, the general principle is clear and acceptable.

These problems become more acute when we consider the international dimension of health. In a developed country like the United Kingdom international aspects have several implications. The first relates to communicable disease, and with the ease of transport now the possibility of transmission to different populations becomes ever easier. Movement for business, leisure, or migration of populations is occurring on a scale as never before. The great plague, cholera and influenza epidemics of the past, and AIDS, tuberculosis and malaria in the present, show just how vulnerable the world is to such infections. The introduction of quarantine in Italy and France, in the 14th century, was one of the earliest attempts to control infections, and there is still ethical justification for certain sorts of boundary control for health reasons.

The need for international legislation is apparent also if we consider environmental issues, the most recent and serious of which was the radioactive release in Chernobyl. But environmental problems regularly cross international boundaries as the effects of acid rain and global warming make clear. The need to ensure that there is an environmental impact assessment of economic growth has been set out in a series of programmes of 'sustainable development'.

Legislation and Health Promotion

Has the state any justification for using fiscal policy for passing legislation to promote positive health or well-being? A strong argument for maintaining that a government does have a duty to promote positive health can be found in the preamble to the Constitution of WHO (1946), which asserts that there is a right to positive health. In ambitious terms it states: 'The enjoyment of the highest attainable standard of health is one of the fundamental rights of every human being without distinction of race, religion, political belief, economic or social condition.' If this is a fundamental right, then presumably there is a correlative duty laid upon governments to implement it. In other words, acceptance of the WHO Constitution commits states to health and welfare policies. How far such policies can be implemented no doubt turns on the wealth of the country, but there can be no doubt that wealthy Western nations are committed to implementing fiscal and legislative policies to enhance positive health.

To argue that there is a duty on governments to promote health for its own sake still leaves some questions unanswered. Supposing there is such a duty, can it be implemented other than at the expense of individual autonomy?

It is easy to slip into the error of regarding all legislation on the model of the criminal law — as restrictive prohibition backed by sanction. But this is an oversimplified way of looking at some health legislation. For example, legislation may require public bodies to make provision for the disabled. This is more aptly seen as positive creation of new opportunities than as negative prohibition. There are legal requirements on factory owners to restrict unpleasant pollutants, and on car manufacturers to ensure certain safety standards. Indeed, there is an enormous range of health legislation with a positive slant. Whereas this may diminish the freedom of some groups in society, it certainly extends the freedom of the majority and improves their quality of life (Pinet, 1987).

If we think of autonomy in this way, then health legislation is not *removing* our individual autonomy but rather *enhancing* it. In improving the general quality of life, legislation can add to our autonomy. This is obviously the case if we consider the example of provision for the disabled, but it is true also of anti-pollution legislation and many other types of health legislation.

Legislation and Citizenship

So far in this section we have been concerned with the role of the state and health legislation. But there is much more to the 'organised efforts of society' than legislation. Let us state the five principles which the WHO (1984) sees as the basis of health promotion:

1. Health promotion involves the population as a whole in the context of their everyday life, rather than focusing on people at risk for specific diseases.

2. Health promotion is directed towards action on the causes or determinants of health.
3. Health promotion combines diverse, but complementary methods or approaches, including communication, education, legislation, fiscal measures, organisational change, community development and spontaneous local activities against health hazards.
4. Health promotion aims particularly at effective and concrete public participation.
5. While health promotion is basically an activity in the health and social fields, and not a medical service, health professionals — particularly in primary health care — have an important role in nurturing and enabling promotion.

How are we to interpret phrases such as 'concrete public participation'? What is the ethical importance of this approach?

One way of making sense of this idea is to think of society not in terms of the individuals who make it up, but in terms of the institutions, practices, customs, political arrangements, and social class relationships which give structure to the society. From this point of view, people are related to each other by the structures of their society, and indeed part of their identity is created by these social structures. We could then evaluate a society in terms of the way in which its social structures tend to produce health in the people who belong to that society. Just as we sometimes praise the 'atmosphere' in a school or hospital as one of well-being, so the social structures of an entire society might be said to make for or detract from health or well-being.

Some theorists with firm attachments to individualism might prefer to understand what we have said as referring to health determinants rather than health itself. For example, they might agree that a society with marked social class gradients and corresponding gradients in the distribution of ill-health is one with a tendency to create ill-health in individuals. Thus, in terms of this approach, if we speak of an 'unhealthy society' we are simply speaking metaphorically about the determinants, such as poor housing and diet and so on, that have helped to produce poor health states in individuals. Other thinkers might be prepared to extend language and to maintain that it is not a metaphor to characterise social relationships and structures as being themselves unhealthy. It is perhaps self-indulgent to pursue this theoretical question here, but it is certainly one way of making sense of the phrase 'the organised efforts of society', in the Acheson Report (1988), or 'effective and concrete public participation', as the WHO principle puts it (1984).

One context in which these phrases may have more practical meaning is that of rationing. We have already touched on this issue in terms of the debate over resource allocation in primary and secondary care. There now seems to be a movement — famously initiated in the State of Oregon (Smith, 1996) — to involve the public in decisions about rationing health care resources. One example of this is the use of 'citizens' juries' in the Cambridge and Huntingdon Health Authority (Lenaghan *et al.*, 1996). In a pilot scheme a group of local people were recruited and met for 4 days to consider how priorities for rationing health care should be set and how far the public should be involved in these decisions. The discussions were mainly on matters of process but the project indicated a willingness amongst the public to be involved in matters of priority setting.

To the extent that there is exclusive emphasis on state delivery of health care to individuals, there is the invitation to see health as a commodity to be supplied by the state. The same is true if we think of health as a commodity bought by private health insurance. But health is not in any sense a commodity. Health and well-being are, in the end, a set of relationships among citizens and the involvement of citizens in decisions about rationing is a good example. As Beauchamp (1987 p.72) wrote:

Collective goods are ultimately a set of relationships among the citizens of a community, relationships in which the community as a whole participates to obtain desired benefits. These collective goods include aggregate states of welfare or well-being, including declining rates of disease and premature deaths; efforts to limit the resources society devotes to personal health services; shared and common access to a good like medical care to foster the sense of community and membership in the group itself. And finally, there are those highly important collective goods, shared or common beliefs and values.

It is clear that we can add a legal system to Beauchamp's list, and in particular one designed to stimulate social responsibility. Indeed, it is plausible to suggest that the increasing government intervention on drunk-driving issues has encouraged a greater social awareness about the dangers of alcohol more generally, and thus a greater sense of community and individual responsibility. In a similar way, legislation designed to assist disabled or handicapped persons can also increase a sense of community responsibility for those groups. In other words, in so far as health legislation and other governmental health policies are directed at increasing community awareness, as distinct from being directed at the good of specific individuals, it is not paternalistic.

A health alliance which has been shown to be helpful in developing community awareness is that between health promotion ser-

PUBLIC HEALTH AND ETHICS 267

vices and community arts. Several projects have taken place and
have had favourable evaluations. For example, the Bristol Area
Specialist Health Promotion Service report on these projects: pho-
tography, the visual arts and drama (Hecht, 1996). Again, Bromley
by Bow have on-going community arts and health projects
(Bromley By Bow Centre, 1995). The central message from these
and similar projects is that disease and ill-health cannot be eradi-
cated by narrowly medical means; they must be tackled in a community context with the approval of the community. In other
words, medicine needs health alliances, and the arts are a vital and
ethically acceptable ally. The ancient Greeks recognised this when
they made Apollo god of both medicine and the arts.

CONCLUSIONS

It is often assumed that ethical problems in medicine are the prerog-
ative of clinical practice, and that the problems of public health medicine are those of public policy and legislation. But we have tried to
bring out that the policies advocated by public health medicine do
indeed raise ethical issues of a basic kind involving principles of justice, utility and individual rights. Moreover, these familiar ethical
concepts must be supplemented by some which are less familiar. If
the collective goods which are promoted by public health medicine
are to be achieved, the methods must involve the development of
community identity and awareness. In other words, public health
medicine, to be effective in an ethically acceptable manner, must seek
health alliances with other community movements.

REFERENCES

Acheson Report 1988 Public Health in England. Report of the Commitee of
    Inquiry into the future development of the public health function. HMSO,
    London
Beauchamp D 1987 Lifestyle, public health and paternalism. In Ethical Dilemmas
    in Health Promotion. ed S Dioxiadis. John Wiley, Chichester
Blaney R 1987 Why Prevent Disease? In Ethical Dilemmas in Health Promotion
    ed S Dioxiadis. John Wiley, Chichester
Bogle I, Chisholm J 1996 Primary care: restoring the jewel in the crown British
    Medical Journal, editorial 312: 1624–5
Bromley By Bow Centre Annual Report 1995–6 Bromley by Bow, London
British Medical Journal 1996 News Section 313: 1424
Calman KC, Downie RS 1997 Ethical principles and ethical issues in public health.
    In Oxford Textbook of Public Health vol 1 Oxford University Press, Oxford
Charlton B 1993 Public health medicine — a different kind of ethics? Journal of
    the Royal Society of Medicine 86: 194–5

Department of Health 1992 The Health of the Nation: A strategy for England. HMSO, London

Department of Health 1996 Primary Care: The future, choice and opportunity. HMSO, London

Department of Health and Human Services, Public Health Service 1991 Healthy People: National health promotion and disease prevention objectives. US Government Printing Office, Washington DC

Downie RS, Tannahill C, Tannahill A 1996 Health Promotion: Models and values. 2nd edn. Oxford University Press, Oxford

Hecht R ed 1996 I Talk Now. Bristol Specialist Health Promotion Service, Central Health Clinic, Bristol

Hermanson B, Omenn GS, Kronmal RA, Gersh BJ 1988 Beneficial six-year outcome of smoking cessation in older men and women with coronary artery disease New England Journal of Medicine 319: 1365–9

Kammerling RM, Kinnear A 1996 The extent of the two tier service for fundholders British Medical Journal 312: 1399–401

Kelly MP, Charlton B 1992 Health promotion: time for a new philosophy? British Journal of General Practice, editorial 223–4

Knox EG 1987 Personal and public health care: conflict, congruence or accommodation? In Ethical Dilemmas in Health Promotion. ed. S Dioxiadis JohnWiley, Chichester

Lenaghan J, New B, Mitchell E 1996 Setting priorities: is there a role for citizens' juries? British Medical Journal 312: 1553–4

Omenn GS 1990 Prevention and the elderly: what are appropriate policies? Health Affairs 9: 80–93

Pinet G 1987 Health legislation, prevention and ethics. In Ethical Dilemma in Health Promotion ed. S. Dioxiadis, John Wiley, Chichester

Report of the working party on fluoridation of water and cancer 1985 A review of the epidemiological evidence 1985 HMSO, London

Roland M 1996 Defining core general practitioner services: a threat to the future of general practice. British Medical Journal 313: 704

Shickle D, Chadwick R 1994 The ethics of screening: is 'screeningitis' an incurable disease? Journal of Medical Ethics 20: 12–18

Smith R 1996 Rationing health care: moving the debate forward. British Medical Journal, editorial 312: 1553–4

Stewart-Brown S, Gillam S, Jewell T 1996 The problems of fundholding British Medical Journal, editorial 312: 1311–2

Stone D, Stewart S 1994 Towards a screening strategy for Scotland. Scottish Forum for Public Health Medicine, Glasgow

Tones BK, Tilford S 1994 Health Education: Effectiveness and efficiency. Chapman and Hall, London

Walters L 1988 Ethical issues in the prevention and treatment of HIV infection and AIDS. Science 239: 597–603

Whitehead M 1987 The Health Divide: Inequalities in health in the 1980s. Health Education Council, London

Whitehead M 1990 The Concepts and Principles of Equity and Health. WHO European Regional Office

Williams G 1984 HealthPromotion — caring concern or slick salesmanship? Journal of Medical Ethics 10: 191–5

World Health Organisation (WHO) 1946 Constitution. WHO, New York

WHO 1984 Health Promotion: a discussion document on the concepts and principles. WHO, Copenhagen

15. Public Health: An organised multi-disciplinary effort

Klim McPherson and John Fox in collaboration with Sheila Adam, Yvonne Cornish, Jenny Griffiths, Teri Knight and Lillian Sommervaille of the Multi-Disciplinary Public Health Forum

INTRODUCTION

That public health is intrinsically multi-disciplinary is obvious. The health of populations is clearly a matter of understanding about health, but also about populations. It is about the complex interaction of individual health and health concerns with the broad and intricate features of populations; their social, political and economic reality. That this needs to be stated at all is an unhappy consequence of one particular social reality; the desire of particular groups to exert a dominance over other groups for their own advantage.

The practice of public health in the UK is to be understood in its historical context, which itself is complex. This is because society has changed, medical technology has changed, health beliefs have changed and the role of professions have changed; all in complicated and diverse ways, since public health became a conscious issue in public policy. In particular, the perceived role of public health has dramatically changed as the old problems of infectious disease have been superseded by the new problems of chronic disease — with dominant behavioural and political components to aetiology, now to the newer highly complex problems of communicable disease, CJD and AIDS, not to mention *E.coli* infection. It has a legitimate remit which must transcend sectoral boundaries and is as important in agriculture, for example, as it is in the health service. The public health agenda is widening, especially in the inner urban environment and is failing to reach crucial Health of the Nation targets.

For a long time, until around the 1920s, engineers were relatively dominant in public health, because it was considered the expertise most appropriate to the effective maintenance of the publics' health.

The dominant model of the 19th century attributed little importance to medicine in preventing disease. Acheson described the response to the cholera epidemics, when a Central Board of Health had been formed in the 1830s (Acheson, 1990) This consisted of 12 members, of whom seven were physicians, but this degree of medical control was questioned by both Edwin Chadwick and the Lancet.

Chadwick was an upwardly mobile lawyer, according to Dorothy Porter, and a disciple of Jeremy Bentham, the founder of the Utilitarian school of classical political economy (Porter, 1996). He had written on cholera prevention, that 'aid must be sought from the Civil Engineer, not from the physician who has done his work when he has pointed out the disease that results from the neglect of proper administrative measures, and he has alleviated the suffering of his victim'(Chadwick, 1842).

The Lancet too was critical of the medical members of the Central Board of Health writing in an 1831 editorial that they were 'drones, sycophants, courtiers and titled imbecility'(Anon, 1981), a different kind of criticism than that of Chadwick. In a circumstance where the practical and scientific underpinning for the prevention (of cholera) was poorly understood, the room for professional, as opposed to scientific, manoeuvring was great. The Privy Council, influenced by Chadwick, dissolved the Board, and formed another of which none of the members were medical. There was to be an advisory committee of physicians, should information about medical matters be required. Perhaps the enduring irony was that the previous Board attracted a grant to each member of £500 while members of the new committee attracted no remuneration.

Nowadays, in similar circumstances of scientific uncertainty affecting the much broader public health concerns, the practice of public health is still plagued, indeed dominated, by professional, sectoral and disciplinary rivalries. Just as in the 19th century the medicalisation of public health reduced the engineers to support staff, so today public health medicine has, until recently, had considerable success in reducing public health social scientists, statisticians, biologists, economists and others to mere support staff (NHS Executive, 1995).

PUBLIC HEALTH MEDICINE

The history of this process is well known; notwithstanding the clear perception[1] of broadly based scientific public health needs, the

---

[1] This clear perception is illustrated both by the FPHM training programmes and by the highly successful research endeavours discussed annually at the scientific meeting of SSM.

Faculty of Community Medicine, later to become the Faculty of Public Health Medicine (FPHM) had created itself in 1972 with exclusive Standing Orders, accommodating only medically qualified people to train for the only professional qualification in public health, while emphasising its strong links with the Royal College of Physicians (Warren, 1996). The concern for historical reasons, largely the move of John Ryle from the Regius chair of Physic at Cambridge to the first Chair of Social Medicine at Oxford in 1942, was not unnaturally to emphasise the links between preventive medicine and clinical medicine. But there are obviously other equally strong links with engineers, social scientists, nurses and statisticians.

The establishment in 1976 of wide-ranging training consortia throughout the country enabled multidisciplinary teaching for medically qualified trainees. The longstanding availability of exclusive MSc courses in epidemiology and public health medicine, consolidated the division in training opportunities between those medically qualified and those who were not. Of course during the 20 to 30 years that these courses were available, there have been a minority which were not limited to medically qualified candidates. However, wanting to do such a course in the absence of funding, or any coherent career structure, was unusual. During the period since 1972, systematic opportunities and funding for 'non-medical' training in public health have not existed, thus consolidating the increasing hegemony of the FPHM and medically qualified public health. This had been further cast in concrete by the generous funding (related to a solid career structure) of trainees in PHM over some 25 years, from NHS training budgets, which usually included salaries, fees and travel allowances. These could not compare with occasional opportunities for bursaries in unusual circumstances for very few students in other disciplines. Since the late 1980s all these courses are open, but funding and career opportunities remain very unequal. (Jefferys & Lashoff, 1991).

It has been estimated that training costs for trainees in PHM are approximately £25,000 per annum, £100,000 per trainee. At the London School of Hygiene alone around 15 students in PHM a year are funded by the NHS and a couple more by other Government Departments and have been since the early 1970s. On top of this, the MSc in Epidemiology attracts another 15 or so students, which, until very recently, were exclusively medical and funded in large measure by MRC or Wellcome. This represents a significant investment in training for a particular group, the exclusivity of which cannot be (or at least has never been convincingly) justified and whose dominance is increasingly irrelevant to the contemporary public health needs of populations.

During this time, representations of various kinds have been made to enhance the training opportunities for 'non medical' people in public health. It had seemed odd that much of the teaching for PHM has been the responsibility of 'non medical' academic colleagues precisely because PHM, even as practised, is unambiguously a multi-disciplinary endeavour. The problems have been twofold; first the unavailability of 'non-medical' training budgets for a training function deemed to be well, and expensively, provided for by PHM training. Secondly, of course, the FPHM (directly or indirectly) has systematically resisted greater autonomy of the 'non-medical' teachers and training programmes and certainly, until very recently, any use of NHS public health training budgets for 'non-medical' training needs. The belief is simply that public health is a medical specialty.

The 1988 enquiry into the Public Health Function chaired by Sir Donald Acheson consolidated the process of securing a separate place for public health within the health service. While the public health function was readily acknowledged to be inter-disciplinary, this merely reinforced the accepted belief that the training in public health (medicine) should therefore be multi-disciplinary. But cleverly the very wording of the role consolidated the real separation. Importantly, what emerged was the recommendation that the name of the specialty should change from Community Medicine to Public Health Medicine.

The slightly gratuitous redundancy in the term 'Public Health Medicine' is unexceptional as a description of a medical specialty of course. But it implies further that the medical model for public health is embraced by the term and that public health (when not taken as simply synonymous with public health medicine), as it might otherwise be practised, embraces other models. This is accentuated by the consequent growth of the description 'non-medical' practitioners of public health (meaning people not qualified in medicine) which implies non-medical assumptions. For people who have spent their whole professional lives working in medical schools concerned with matters of health, who are certainly not 'non-medical', to be routinely referred to as 'non-medical' is just incorrect, whether they accept the dominant tenets of the medical model or not.

The often repeated slogan during the 1970s and 1980s that public health medicine was 'that medical specialty that dealt with the health of populations' served largely to identify the insecurity of a professional group many of whom felt marginalised by their peers and illustrated the desire to emphasise some distinction between it and the rest of public health. The distinction is first obvious but secondly not necessarily of any profound importance, or if it is, it has not been fully explained. The organisation of public health has not been well served by these insecurities, firstly because of the gratuitous division, but also because public health research and practice requires a dispassionate and equal perception of all possible contributing forces affecting the publics' health. To be obviously and institutionally deferential to one sector, albeit a highly important one, must compromise this balance. Unfortunately, public health medicine itself is also discredited by such insecurities.

However, with the inexorable growth of the importance of other disciplines in public health the term is now becoming increasingly limited, rather than limiting. For a long time public health essentially was, at least institutionally, public health medicine, but increasingly public health medicine is becoming but a part of public health, which is what it is. Hence public health medicine used to claim public health, the rest being statisticians or economists or sociologists interested in (and contributing to) public health. However, the Faculty of Public Health Medicine has recently suggested the creation, to celebrate its 25 years, of a Public Health Policy Unit, without any proper involvement with other public health professions. It still has to be pointed out to them that such an idea as proposed would be problematic. Apparently they do now recognise that a Public Health Medicine Policy Unit would not be quite so attractive for charitable funding. And as we shall discuss below the significant development of institutional public health for the public's health requires collaboration by and with the Faculty.

ACADEMIC PUBLIC HEALTH

Because the academic pursuit of public health has always required considerable expertise in several core disciplines, it has always been multidisciplinary, although the 'officer' class were traditionally medically qualified. Only since the late 1980s were professors of public health, for instance, allowed to be people qualified in subjects other than medicine. This has been the source of major tension between public health professionals. However the salary scales remain totally different, largely because (according to the BMA) parity with service colleagues is a principle of much greater importance than parity with academic colleagues. Not to trivialise the point, while it is clear that the practice of surgery should encompass economic, methodological and social considerations, such matters are peripheral to such practice, and surgery is dominant. In these circumstances, parity with NHS colleagues is vital (but not realised because of contractual differences in the opportunities for private practice, of course). Public health, on the other hand, cannot effectively proceed at all without detailed knowledge of the social and statistical sciences as well as the application of medicine. The appropriate peer groups have always been obvious.

The problem for public health has always been the perceived dominance of single disciplines (engineering or medicine, for example) in an intellectual enterprise of many disciplines which can be seen as marginal to the main thrust of each. Public health actually embraces several core disciplines, each of which is ancillary to the main purpose and none of which is obviously dominant. If it is epidemiology, as many suggest (originally of course Jerry Morris (1969)), then people originally trained in many quantitative disciplines can be, and are, excellent epidemiologists. However, the dominant recent tradition in the UK and in Europe that public health departments should be part of medical schools automatically furthers the illusion that medicine is the dominant discipline.

An important contribution that has resulted from the tendency to establish medicine as the dominant tradition in public health have been the attempts to make social medicine central among medical specialities (Lewis, 1991). A long tradition exemplified again by Ryle in Oxford was to assert the key role of public health and social medicine to applied aetiology. Ryle wrote in 1942

social medicine is clinical medicine activated in its aetiological enquiries by social conscience as well as scientific interest and having its main purpose the education of progressive and lay thought and the direction of legislation on behalf of national health and efficiency (Ryle, 1942).

In order to pursue this objective of emphasising the role of social medicine to clinical medicine, two separate things had to happen. The first was to maintain a strong academic respectability, and secondly it was necessary to constrain the concept of public health to keep it well within the legitimate orbit of medical endeavour.

Most departments of social and community medicine in Europe have had to struggle anyway to carve a scientific and academic identity and an appropriate place in traditional single disciplinary surroundings. Thus any such department has had to accommodate a serious dialectical historical process, and struggle to achieve its appropriate structure and position. Clinical medicine thus tends to claim an illegitimate dominance in the concepts of public health, thus emphasising biology, which can itself turn the other constituent disciplines centred outside medicine against the interests of social medicine or public health. The implications are usually variable across settings and not at all stationary with time.

Thus these departments have emerged from the social medicine traditions of the 1940s into what often looks like a pragmatic compromise between what was available and what was desirable. That is the historical tradition of these departments, often with bequeathed academic positions (obviously strongly medical), joint experience and a set of (changing) implied objectives have been combined together with the individual enthusiasms of those staff. Neither the University structures, nor possibly the national research funding structures, were generally well placed to encourage a more directed, principled approach to the structuring of public health in academia. Such an approach would have created Schools of Public Health, rather like the US tradition or similar to business schools, which were autonomous and able to build a truly multidisciplinary faculty. In such circumstance the central concerns of public health and the true scientific uncertainties might have dominated the development more than ancillary desires to achieve professional or disciplinary hegemony.

Such processes have been common throughout Europe (WHO, 1996) and are in different stages of development in different places. They epitomise the emerging role of public health as a crucial science which has, surprisingly to many, but one foot in the medical milieu. The other feet sometimes lack the confidence to stand where they should, possibly because of perceived medical dominance or because of important structural and historical constraints. But 'social medicine' none the less has a theoretical and empirical underpinning, quite as important for public health, in the social and statistical sciences. Moreover the legitimate responsibilities for professional public health are not at all restricted to the health sector.

What we observe are departments concentrating their work on various themes of classical social medicine. This often represents a strong and broad infrastructure from which to grasp the opportunities available to these departments. However, the organisational responsibilities associated with expanding departments, combined with significant extra teaching after Todd in 1968 and other commitments often compromise the clear need to develop a more coherent research structure concentrating on academic excellence, and the true complexities of contemporary public health. All the time the pressures alluded to above tended to have the effect of sacrificing 'social epidemiology' for 'clinical epidemiology', to put it very simply. More recently, of course, 'statistical' epidemiology has achieved a dominance even surpassing that of clinical epidemiology.

However, the emergence, in the UK, of a more dominant R&D function in the NHS has significantly changed the direction and determinants of academic research in public health, towards a more relevant and sceptical scientific model, clearly involving many disciplines as equals. The role of the European Commission on public health practice is also very important in this process, because it encourages collaborative research into issue of public health across Europe. The European Public Health Association (EUPHA) is beginning now to consolidate these collaborations by holding successful annual scientific meetings across Europe, as defined by the WHO. Also the changing political climate, and indeed the persuasiveness of the evidence, has also been important in (re)-legitimising social medicine (Wilkinson, 1996). This has meant that the role of 'non-medical' public health professionals is inevitably promoted. It also means that, for the first time, systematic and directed emphasis is applied to the needs of groups of researchers into health and health services, who are themselves often truly multi-disciplinary.

Whatever effect all of this history has on individuals currently researching or practising in public health from a variety of disciplines, one key implication is that bright graduates from disciplines other than medicine will tend not to choose public health as a career. Moreover, the nature of public health itself, in the medical context, also means that bright medical graduates, unless possessed of a singular determination to practice as social, epidemiological or quantitative medical scientists, will be unlikely to choose public health as a career on its intrinsic merits. Clearly, there will always be significant exceptions to these aggregate tendencies, but this is none the less a real double jeopardy. One group will tend to avoid a support role to a medical specialty and the other a non-clinical role to a clinical profession. Thus public health will remain marginal to both until it can unite into a single scientific function.

THE SOCIETY FOR SOCIAL MEDICINE

The role of the Society for Social Medicine (SSM) has been crucial in the collaborative development of academic public health. The

Society has offered the only truly multi-disciplinary, and scientific, forum for discussion and presentation of research findings at its annual scientific meetings. With more than 1000 members from all disciplines, but deficient in economists, the main activity is between relatively junior public health researchers often presenting their research for the first time in a full programme of diverse results. Most of the participants at the annual scientific meeting are from academic departments of public health, many of whom, of course, are the people who have for many years been engaged in the multi-disciplinary training in public health medicine. However, it traditionally finds questions of actual public health policy, and particularly of professional and educational policy, difficult to deal with. This reflects its Constitution but also must, in part, reflect the ambiguous attitude of the Society to the formation of the Faculty in 1972 and the very iniquitous provision of training, support and career opportunities in the years since its formation. The consequent tensions, while mostly not expressed, can only be exacerbated by such discussion.

In the discussions that led to the creation of the Faculty a working party (consisting of ten public health doctors) had in the autumn of 1969 made a 'Proposal' to guide its formation (Warren, 1996). This had proposed specifically:

- a new organisation with
- the objectives of promoting high standards of training and practice. Its membership would
- be restricted to registered medical practitioners but that later, with the agreement of Royal Colleges, consideration would be given to others engaged in academic community medicine.

Some opposition to these proposals was voiced at an extraordinary general meeting of the Society in June 1970. Apparently 56 people attended of which only 6 were not medically qualified. The opposition came from Margot Jefferys who thought that the exclusion of social scientists would be divisive and would reflect adversely on their status in their academic departments. She also felt that the association with the Royal Colleges would inevitably shift the emphasis of social medicine away from population studies towards social epidemiology. She was concerned too that the creation of the Faculty would alter the function of the Society.

A ballot of members of the Society was conducted by Margot Jefferys and Ann Cartwright. Of the 214 listed members some 67% favoured the formation of a Faculty and 75% favoured the inclusion of non-medically qualified members. If people who were not medically qualified were to be excluded, only 44% of the members favoured such a move; 47% of the medically qualified members. Thus the Society was clearly pressing for a Faculty which concerned itself with education and training for public health, and the maintenance of high standards, but which was multidisciplinary.

However the lure of a Fellowship of the Royal Colleges of Physicians was too much for the Medical Officers of Health, who generally felt undervalued by their clinical colleagues, and cared little for the academic niceties of multi-disciplinary social medicine. Of course, such a prize was not to be anyway, as the Colleges pretty smartly rejected any such proposal. The Faculty had to award its own Fellowships which, scandalously to many, are still only open to medically qualified practitioners of public health.

THE PRACTICE OF PUBLIC HEALTH IN THE UK

The 1974 social reforms separated local government responsibilities for the environment, education and housing from health authorities and the delivery of health care. Then subsequently, with the introduction of managed units and then trusts, the provider aspects of public health within the NHS became increasingly fragmented and distanced from public health departments within health authorities. Most recently, the new thrust for a primary-care-led NHS both promotes and detracts from a public health perspective — with GPs increasingly aware (Hart, 1988) of their practices as populations, but singularly untrained and poorly equipped to deal systematically with the public health issues. At the same time public health nurses (as a result of the culture of contract-based contracting) are increasingly focusing on individual patients within practices and less on their populations. However, the internal market should increase the need for public health skills.

But the position of public health on the purchasing side remains ambiguous, and concentrates on rationalising clinical services. Public Health can promote the broader role of health authorities, in their main responsibility for the population's health, by engaging in issues outside the health care contracting culture and including the incorporation of relevant issues of environment, housing and education. But, there is the problem of the real effectiveness of public health advocacy (which is dominated by public health medicine, for the reasons discussed) and corporate managerial responsibility.

Public health is divided between professional and disciplinary allegiances in a very profound and serious way.

A common argument made by public health doctors stresses that this effectiveness is greater when public health is seen to be largely a medical specialty, with medical leadership. This is an argument which seeks to justify the status quo described above, but has no obvious justification apart from an appeal to a lay view of public health which might sometimes just assume that public health is a medical specialty. The actual contribution of the (collaborative) work of other disciplines to the theory and effective practice of public health is also dominant. Not to speak of Florence Nightingale and Bradford Hill and many others, one has only to leaf through the pages of the *BMJ* or the *Lancet* to discover papers whose practical implications for public health knowledge are profound. Then, if one is really interested in pursuing such distinctions, the original discipline of instigators and executors of such work can be seen to be obviously multi-disciplinary.

A false linkage between responsibility and professional identity then is likely to give rise to division between those engaged in the practice of public health, with consequent fragmentation across the divides of trusts and the primary/secondary care interface. Clearly, also a dominant group a part of which seeks some of its credibility from its affinity to clinical medicine and individual patients may well have problems separating these concerns from their responsibility for the population's health.

Of course, it is currently a statutory requirement that Directors of public health should be medically qualified. In other countries, Australia for instance, the detrimental effect such a policy has on the career and morale of other aspiring public health practitioners is blunted by appointing to the top public health jobs on merit, not discipline, and requiring that appropriate medical responsibility is held by an appointee at senior level. Clearly, to train for public health where the most senior appointment must be medically qualified is itself a disincentive. The barriers thus raised between other professional interests in health and in these related services, among those committed to the population perspective, make working together more difficult.

THE ORGANISATION OF PUBLIC HEALTH IN THE UK

Public health is clearly organised around the dominance of medically qualified public health practitioners. All of the 2000 or so accredited professionals in public health are trained in public health medicine. They are automatically senior to other practitioners of scientific public health (although not necessarily to managers), and organise themselves around various formal and informal networks. These networks until very recently were almost exclusively for medically qualified practitioners. Directors of public health tend to meet regularly and the CMO of England chairs a national public health network which is predominantly composed of medically qualified people. Regional public health meetings are variable, some being advertised within the Faculty structure while others are becoming consciously multi-disciplinary. But progress is inevitably slow and few of the transforming initiatives have yet come spontaneously from public health medicine.

Public health consists of several disciplines, each ancillary to public health, which are complementary. First, from the point of view of the disciplines, public health is but one part of their concern and is likely to be disparaged by purists in the discipline (Strong, 1979), particularly if dominated by another. Second, this gives rise to a seemingly inevitable quest for a dominance of public health from individual disciplines, with claims justified by their own perception of what is important in public health. With the real uncertainties facing effective public health policy, and the formidable difficulties associated with its evaluation, the room for irrefutable claims of legitimate hegemony is just too great. And, once the consequences are consolidated they develop a formidable momentum, particularly if they have an obvious and simple appeal. Public health is after all about health.

However, public health is too important, and too difficult, to allow this silliness to continue. Whatever we do not know about the public's health, we certainly know that the organisation of public health does little justice to its importance. The need for coherent and effective public health advocacy and the urgent need for strong and united public health leadership is widely acknowledged. Institutional public health is essentially dysfunctional in contemporary Britain.

Public health is organised in a manner reflecting past unjustified assumptions of appropriate power. It has failed to develop adequate obvious public health functions. These functions should be essentially:

- the statutory function;
- an effective public health umbrella function, including possibly a public health advocacy function;
- various professional functions;
- an academic function; and

- single issue advocacy functions represented commonly by NGOs.

Whereas the professional functions are obviously important; they must be subordinated to strategies and objectives clearly justifiable in terms of the public's health. The professional needs of particular groups have to be seen clearly to have a public health purpose. While this hope is naïve, such justification ought to be formally made every time particular claims are made or the consequence of past established special interests noted.

Meanwhile public health will remain divided while one disci pline claims any unjustified dominance. Thus public health, in present circumstances, cannot organise any legitimate leadership nor any advocacy role which will not be seen as, and be, both partisan and weak. Indeed many key figures in public health distance themselves from the enterprise since it is seen to be thus restricted, hijacked or abused. These circumstances also tend to mean that public health is too closely tied to the health service at the expense of other areas of important public policy, and too closely allied with various health service management functions. Public health in the UK is thus too close to health care and too far from health. This tends to further marginalise the role, and the development, of both scientific public health and multi-disciplinary collaboration.

The requirement for creating an infrastructure which will enable the training and development of a group of accredited professionals in public health, comparable to that which exists for public health medicine, but not so limited, is urgent. The important strategic point is that, since public health is multi-disciplinary, the various professional groups will, in the apparent quest for high quality, seek conditions and resources which will inevitably compete with those sought by other groups in public health. Such claims might be monitored and justified by an effective and representative umbrella organisation, which is lacking in the UK at the moment and is probably essential. There is a need for a structure which can appropriately deal with this phenomenon in a fair and reasonable way. How can public health organisation sensibly move in that direction, while inevitably threatening several vested interests?

TAKING THE ORGANISATION OF PUBLIC HEALTH FORWARD.

Unquestionably the dominant force in public health strategy in the UK is, *de facto*, the Faculty of Public Health Medicine, because of its success in creating a large cadre (2000 plus) of well-trained professionals in established (and important) positions in the Health Service. This, however, is unfortunate because they themselves mostly regard themselves as weak relative to their regular comparators, the clinicians and the Royal Colleges. But they are strong relative to public health sociologists, for example.

Because the increasing need for more appropriate organisational structures exerted pressure on the Faculty during the 1980s and 1990s, it had created a category of Honorary Members in 1991. These people were nominated and elected on some criteria of merit in public health and were not medically qualified. They pay (paradoxically) a subscription to the Faculty and have limited rights in the Faculty structure. However, since the Standing Orders of the Faculty clearly restrict it to pursuing the interests of public health medicine, it has always been difficult to see what the point of (costly) Honorary Membership actually was. Honorary Members are represented on the various Faculty Committees, but since the purpose is so restricted it is difficult to see how busy people would spend time on it, particularly since, at least until now, the effect is inevitably to constrain, certainly not enhance, opportunities in other branches of public health. However, recently, the Honorary Members have been allowed two members on the Board, and one on the Executive. This is useful because at least the most unjustifiable special interest and sectional claims, whether or not in the name of high standards, can be questioned, if not sensibly dealt with.

In 1994 the Faculty of Public Health Medicine commissioned a postal survey of public health professionals from backgrounds other than medicine. This survey was designed firstly to identify as many of this previously undescribed group as possible, and then to build a picture of the training and career needs of the group (Faculty of Public Health Medicine, 1995). Over 1000 individuals were identified whose training and career prospects were at best *ad hoc*. More worryingly, from the perspective of developing effective multi-disciplinary working, it was often non-existent. Over half had no formal training in public health and of these only a half had received funding for such training. Respondents frequently felt unrecognised, undervalued and inequitably treated and many were not members of any public health organisation.

The survey was followed by a one-day workshop based meeting held in Birmingham in January 1995, where the issues concerned with career structure, training, accreditation and professional roles and responsibilities were explored in more depth. This was the beginning of the Multi-Disciplinary Public Health Forum.

In 1995, the Public Health Medicine Faculty Board took a bold decision to encourage a multi-disciplinary agenda for training and accreditation in public health, as well as full membership of the Faculty itself. This revisited the quite deliberate discussions in the early 1970s, when the Faculty was created, which accommodated the possibility of a multi-disciplinary faculty. The proposal was to allow people trained in relevant disciplines other than medicine to take Faculty exams and to allow membership and fellowship of the Faculty on public health qualifications independent of a person's original training. This was in recognition of the intrinsic multi-disciplinary nature of public health policy and practice, and the need for a more co-ordinated and egalitarian activity to establish training and career opportunities for all relevant disciplines in the profession. The notion was that public health was weakened by encouraging disciplinary division and by not exploiting its true diversity.

The Faculty had also conducted a survey to gauge the opinion of members and fellows of the perceived wisdom of opening its membership to guide the AGM of 1996; the response rate was extremely high. Around 52% of 1853 returns agreed that the Faculty should seek to achieve its objectives in terms of public health rather than public health medicine. On the other hand, 54% said that membership of the Faculty should not be opened to non-medics who pass both parts of the MFPHM, while only 39% said that they would wish to see the membership so widened. Clearly, this was a setback for multi-disciplinary public health. Any changes to the Faculty's standing orders would require a three-quarters majority of the AGM, and putting the original Board proposals to the AGM would not have been adequately supported by these results.

Hence the notion of working with the Faculty to pursue the objectives of creating a sensible umbrella organisation is at least clear. The Faculty cannot, since then, be the organisation to do it. The notion, expressed by the ballot, that the Faculty would seek to achieve its objectives in terms of public health rather than public health medicine and at the same time would not want to include other professionals, however well qualified in public health, if they were not medically qualified is worrying. They are no longer in any position to lead public health because of their particular and sectional view of their role in public health and their failure to meet the genuine aspirations of even the medically qualified who want to pursue a population strategy for health gain (Lewis, 1986). But they do have a real responsibility as consequence of their *de facto* role and they could still change if they felt it was important.

It is now clear that the professional development in public health will have to happen separately, and hence the need for separate professional organisation is urgent, whether it should be organised by function, aspiration or by discipline remains to be seen. But with that comes the urgent need to create an umbrella organisation to oversee these activities and to develop the advocacy and leadership functions. This means that training will be split between professions and hence must be separate from a united public health advocacy function. There is a great deal of work to be done by all organisations in public health.

Of course, the Society for Social Medicine is also influential in a very informal way, but under its Constitution has no responsibility for professional or policy concerns. There is also the Association of Public Health (APH) which has a definite multi-disciplinary health service and management advocacy role, which was created in 1992 along the lines of the American Public Health Association (APHA). The APH has at most a few hundred members, while the APHA has 13,000 members representing 77 disciplines in public health and related fields. The APHA tries to be an umbrella organisation whose main areas of activity include setting public health standards, public health education, scientific debate and providing professional opportunities. Advocacy is high on its agenda and networking is integral to the APHA's way of working. Many active interest groups exist, for example, in mental health, in epidemiology, in tobacco and in public health nursing. Interest groups, caucuses and sections meet within the annual conference (attended in 1996 by 13,000 people!), providing opportunities for exchange and development. Effective lobbying is organised by the creation of coalitions of interested groups who can sign up to working together around key issues such as tobacco control, women's health or bioethics.

But the APH in the UK has seen its role as being a public health advocacy organisation which cannot take the development of multi-disciplinary public health forward since it was thought to be too controversial and outside its remit. While not currently a professional organisation it certainly is not barred from changing under direction from its membership, but has recently clearly eschewed any such responsibility.

THE MULTI-DISCIPLINARY PUBLIC HEALTH FORUM

Meanwhile, encouraged by the survey of around 1000 professionals in public health undertaken by the Faculty and by the meeting held

in Birmingham subsequently, another meeting for multi-disciplinary public health was held in April 1996. This had been preceded
by Regional meetings, held in each Region of the UK, to discuss the
professional and other aspects of multi-disciplinary public health
for people not trained in medicine. The meeting in 1996 happened
just as the Faculty ballot and its implications became known.
Indeed, June Crown, the President of the Faculty, spoke about the
role of the Faculty and of her disappointment given that one of her
major goals was to make serious progress on the issue of multi-
disciplinary public health, building on the foundations of her pre-
decessor Michael O'Brien. Her proposal then, in the light of the
results, was to consider the establishment of a College of Public
Health with (possibly) two faculties, one of public health medicine
and the other of public health sciences (possibly). This proposal was
at an early stage in its development and the AGM of the Faculty
decided to conduct a full option appraisal.

The Regional meetings and the meeting in April 1966 were very
successful, and well supported, expressions of a need for some more
formal organisation to pursue some clear common objectives. These
were identified after the regional meetings and further discussion as
follows:

- ensure that the health of the people of the United Kingdom are
  served best by all Public Health Professionals, who are properly
  trained, accredited and developed;
- maintain and build on the diversity of multi-disciplinary public
  health to realise public health goals;
- promote the development of a unified voice for public health
  advocacy;
- promote the development of a single voice for Public Health
  Professionals;
- address the current inequities in training and career opportunities for Public Health Professionals;
- work with the NHS Executive, Public Sector organisations, professional and scientific organisations and employers to further
  these objectives.

The establishment of an interim negotiating group of the Multi-disciplinary Public Health Forum (MDPHF), which would include
the original working party plus representatives of the regional
workshops was agreed. This group would co-opt other members as
appropriate and explore all the options for the further development
of multi-disciplinary public health. The idea would be to report

back to another national meeting in 1997 and to obtain minimal funding to enable appropriate progress. Thus the MDPHF will consider how this new momentum of public health professionals, with a vigorous set of common objectives and ambitions, should dovetail with various public health organisations and opportunities, in some detail. Other organisations are clearly important in the process, in particular other professional and scientific organisations and potential employers; the NHS, local and national, voluntary and government, the education and university sector and elsewhere.

The clear objective is to ensure that the public health interests in the UK are served by the best public health professionals all of whom are properly trained and developed precisely to serve that function. This implies that the MDPHF is concerned about gaps and opportunities in training and development; gaps and opportunities in career development as well as gaps and opportunities in local networking and support. These were the dominant needs identified in the Regional meetings.

To fulfil these objectives, the MDPHF has strengthened the continuing role of regional networks to take forward the aims and objectives of the MDPHF locally as well as nationally. It is establishing an internal and external communication system via: the regional networks and co-ordinating groups and producing a newsletter (The Public Health Forum) circulated to members of regional and local networks with six other interested organisations. It is also assessing the needs for professional development and training using the regional network to promote good practice. It is now beginning to formally assess the requirements of systems for national public health accreditation standards, and will investigate the options for professional integration. In April 1997 it will have investigated and organised options on an action plan to the National Conference of the MDPHF. And, it will investigate means of promoting the aims of the MDPHF in a variety of policy development organisations.

This is happening without any organisational infrastructure with enormous commitment from people who have full time service and academic jobs anyway. The main and most urgent policy item is to try to establish appropriate training budgets for a group of people, for whom the need is difficult to understand by some, while there are consistent underspends in the public health medicine training budgets. Building a new infrastructure when the major strength in unidisciplinary public health is underspent and subject to management cuts and where the wide perception is that public health is a

medical specialty, will certainly not be easy. Not least because per-
force it is a multi-disciplinary programme.

FUNDING FOR EDUCATION AND TRAINING BUDGETS WITHIN THE NHS

The training needs of multi-disciplinary public health must be
tightly related to the nature of multi-disciplinary public health
practice in the future NHS and outside. But even now it is clear that
that funding for training in public health would, in order for it to
be commensurate with that professional need, have to be enhanced.
This will mean more than the *ad hoc* allocation of some of the existing training budgets for 'non-medical' training, but a coherent recommendation for funding a balanced training programme for all
relevant specialties in all appropriate public health functions. The
kind of training that this would entail would clearly involve an
investment in new basic courses in biology and medicine for the
'non-medical' trained candidates and appropriate augmentation of
their disciplinary knowledge with appropriate specialist skills. It
might well look very different from PHM training, taking health
science as the central objective, and hopefully be the better for that.

Proper training infrastructures require adequate champions and
professional models, high quality and available courses related to
service need and often modular approaches to accommodate varying origins. They also require adequate placements and second-
ments, continuing professional development and appraisals as well
as appropriate budgets.

Details of the new arrangements for planning and commissioning non-medical education and training following the abolition of
RHAs were published in an Executive Letter (95)27 in March 1995,
which are now fully operational. A subsequent Executive Letter
contained seven priority areas, one of which was to: *influence the
development of multi-disciplinary education and training.*

From April 1996 funding for education and training is to be met
from three national levies: the R & D levy, the Postgraduate
Medical levy and the Non-Medical Education &Training (NMET)
levy. There is, of course, pressure to reduce, not expand, these levies.
The NMET budgets are now secured by means of a national levy on
all Health Authorities. Most of this money (75%) is already allocated to pre-registration nurse education. Levy requirements for
1996/97 have been determined with a projected total spend of £800
million. In the future the plan is to reduce the NMET budget still

further and rely on consortia to raise local funds and develop local initiatives, particularly with post-graduate training. This clearly has important implications on MDPH which is of necessity arriving late in the process. A key feature of the new arrangements include the establishment of local education consortia. 45 of these consortia have been established across England, varying in size and number in each region. These consortia are made up of representatives from NHS Purchasers and Providers, GPs and GP fund holders together with Social Services and non-NHS providers. These consortia are therefore heavily weighted towards the Trust perspective.

The role of the HAs on the consortia is one of strategic workforce planning to ensure that educational commissioning supports the identified population health needs. However, they are also employers in their own right and so should now be arguing for the development of their own staff as well. Clearly what they perceive as the need for training in multi-disciplinary public health will be crucial. Eventually the consortia will take full responsibility and will place contracts directly with educational providers for training and continuous professional development.

But the possibility for the virement of funds between Post-graduate Medical training budget underspends was lost when the Regional Authorities were formed. Hence multi-disciplinary public health has serious problems in redressing the chronic and long-standing educational funding inequalities in public health, because not only is current funding going to be difficult but there is a great deal of ground to make up too. The need has to be established firmly; while the demand for courses is strong, notwithstanding inadequate funding and poor career prospects.

CONCLUSIONS

The future for public health in the UK is exciting if, and only if, it can concentrate on what it should do; serve the public health needs of the whole community by effectively reducing avoidable ill-health. The most exciting part involves the collaborative development of those components of public health which might have suffered importantly as a consequence of a career structure being attractive only to one discipline. Significant and deliberate development of structures capable of enhancing the opportunities and the careers of those people in public health, for whom an important need can be justified, are required. True intellectual collaboration between disciplines to resolve the complex problems facing public health is an exciting prospect. This means a dispassionate and comprehensive evaluation of that public health need, taking account of possible past inequalities, speculating sensibly about the unexplored possibilities of disciplinary synergy. This probably may require a greater investment in public health itself, to be justified on its estimated benefit to health.

It also means the establishment of an effective umbrella organisation by, and on behalf of, all public health professionals. The professional requirements of all people in public health should be responsive to that need and subordinate to the umbrella organisation, being aware that the opportunities for special pleading are both enormous and boring. They are usually irrelevant to the actual needs of the public's health but only to the needs of the proposers.

The result of the 1997 General Election promises a Minister for Public Health, a new Food Agency and serious health service management cuts, which include public health medicine establishment. The possibility of a serious review of the public health function and a fresh look at public health issues is promised by Tessa Jowell, and we await these initiatives. A question of any health policy for such a minister is the implementation of (belated and) appropriate institutional arrangements for public health in the UK.

Might the creation of a suitably independent National Centre for Public Health, which will be responsible for the maintenance and co-ordination of appropriate evidence based standards, be a sensible solution? Important policy questions in public health to do with priority setting, appropriate screening, secondary and primary prevention strategies, cancer registration and measuring morbidity and health behaviour, for example, are currently resolved in a strangely *ad hoc* manner. Moreover, they necessarily compete with the provision of demand-led clinical services, without any coherent or rational view about the relative effects on health and well-being. All these questions require permanent high-quality systematic contributions to the development and implementation of effective public health programmes. They might benefit from a co-ordinated research and development programme in public health and a greater dedicated contribution to the analysis of national data systems. District Health Authorities, Local Government and Environmental Health Departments, for example, develop public health programmes with much duplication of effort, which are sometimes of mediocre quality. Should such a Centre provide a resource to enable these many devolved organisations to implement programmes based on exploiting available evidence and co-ordinated specialist experience to achieve the best achievable local results? Such an organisation might be the appropriate arbiter of training and accreditation programmes, in collaboration with the Faculty of Public Health Medicine, in public health too.

Even if this is pie in the sky there is little doubt that, under present conditions, multi-disciplinary public health will become much more appropriately institutionalised since it now has a legitimacy, confidence and momentum which is irreversible. It has an expertise which is clearly valuable and many people who are committed to sensible objectives. We end by posing two vital and extremely important conditioning questions without discussion. First, can there be much progress before the Health Service itself disappears into a fragmented privately funded free for all, and secondly, can the vested interests allow it to happen without too much pain? If the answer to both is yes, then we might raise the public profile of scientific public health, develop local networks within our communities and become more capable of influencing the political agenda for public health appropriately. Public health will then be a united and potent force for the public's health which is too long overdue.

ACKNOWLEDGEMENTS

We gratefully acknowledge the sometimes unwitting contribution of ideas from Nick Day, Margot Jefferys, John Powles, Tony McMichael, Sian Griffiths, David Hunter, Fiona Stanley as well as many others. Clearly, they should not be held responsible for any of the more fanciful aspects of this chapter, as indeed should not some of the collaborators themselves.

REFERENCES

Acheson M 1990 The medicalisation of public health; the United Kingsom and the United States contrasted. Journal of Public Health and Medicine 12: 31–8
Anonymous 1831 The Board of Health Lancet ii: 433
Chadwick E 1842 Report on the sanitary condition of the labouring population. London HM Government Report 341
Faculty of Public Health Medicine 1995 The training and career development needs of public health professionals. Report of a survey of professionals in public health. Institute of Environmental Health, University of Birmingham
Hart J D 1988 A new Kind of Doctor. Merlin
Jefferys M, Lashoff J 1991 Preparation for public health: into the twenty-first century. Chapter 9 in Free E & Acheson RM. A History of Education in Public Health. Oxford University Press, Oxford

Lewis J 1986 What price Community Medicine? The philosophy, practice and politics of Public Health since 1919 Wheatsheaf Books, Brighton

Lewis J 1991 The public's health: philosophy and practice in Britain in the twentieth century. In A History of Education in Publlic Health. Eds Fee E & Acheson RM; Oxford

Morris J N 1969 Tomorrow's community physician: Lancet ii: 811–16

NHS Executive 1995 The practice of public health

Porter D 1996 Public health and centralisation: the Victorian British state. Chapter 2. Oxford Textbook of Public Health. Vol. 1 ed R Detels, W Holand, J McEwen, GS Omenn Oxford University Press, Oxford

Ryle J A 1942 Letter British Medical Journal 2801

Strong P 1979 Sociological imperialism and the profession of medicine: a critical examination of the thesis of medical imperialism. Social Science and Medicine 13a: 199–216

The Todd Report 1968 Royal Commission, Report on Medical Education and Training 1865–68 Cmnd 3569. London, HMSO

Warren M 1996 The genesis of the Faculty of Community Medicine. CHSS University of Kent

WHO 1996 European Health Care Reforms; Analysis of Current Strategy. WHO Europe, Copenhagen

Wilkinson R 1996 Unhealthy Societies. Routledge

Index